DANCE THERAPY REDEFINED

DANCE THERAPY REDEFINED
A Body Approach to Therapeutic Dance

By

JOHANNA EXINER

and

DENIS KELYNACK

With

Naomi Aitchison

and

Jenny Czulak

Illustrations by Lisa Roberts

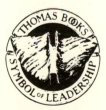

CHARLES C THOMAS • PUBLISHER
Springfield • Illinois • U.S.A.

Published and Distributed Throughout the World by

CHARLES C THOMAS • PUBLISHER
2600 South First Street
Springfield, Illinois 62794-9265

© *1994 by* CHARLES C THOMAS • PUBLISHER
ISBN 0-398-05913-6
Library of Congress Catalog Card Number: 94-8556

With THOMAS BOOKS *careful attention is given to all details of manufacturing
and design. It is the Publisher's desire to present books that are satisfactory as to
their physical qualities and artistic possibilities and appropriate for their particular
use.* THOMAS BOOKS *will be true to those laws of quality that assure a good
name and good will.*

Printed in the United States of America
SC-R-3

Library of Congress Cataloging-in-Publication Data

Exiner, Johanna.
    Dance therapy redefined : a body approach to therapeutic dance /
by Johanna Exiner and Denis Kelynack with Naomi Aitchison and Jenny
Czulak ; illustrations by Lisa Roberts.
        p.   cm.
    Includes bibliographical references and index.
    ISBN 0-398-05913-6
    1. Dance therapy.   I. Kelynack, Denis.   II. Title.
RC489.D3E94   1994
615.8′5155—dc20

94-8556
CIP

ABOUT THE AUTHORS

Johanna Exiner is a graduate of the Academy of Music and the Performing Arts in Vienna, with a major in dance. Her work in the field of movement and dance has branched out in many directions, covering such areas as theatrical, educational and recreational dance and the exploration of dance as a therapeutic medium.

As Senior Lecturer at the Institute of Early Childhood Development in Melbourne, she was instrumental in introducing a Graduate Diploma in Movement and Dance in 1977, the first in Australia and shared in coordinating and teaching in the first Graduate Certificate in Dance Therapy.

Johanna Exiner has conducted regular group sessions in dance therapy at state and private psychiatric institutions.

She has published Teaching Creative Movement and Learning Through Dance with Phyllis Lloyd, and is the author of several papers and articles.

She is a Foundation and Honorary Life Member of the Australian Association for Dance Education, now the Australian Dance Council, and an Associate of the University of Melbourne.

Denis Kelynack is a counselling psychologist in private practice. Before that he was lecturer in psychology at The University of Melbourne and subsequently became a student counsellor there for 20 years. He first studied dance therapy with Tamara Greenberg at the Center for Energetic Studies in Berkeley California. He then completed the Graduate Diploma in Movement and Dance in Melbourne and subsequently taught in that course for six years. He was also teacher with Johanna Exiner in the Grad. Cert. of Dance Therapy at the same institution. He is interested in the relationship of Feldenkrais and Alexander techniques to dance therapy and has had experience of both of these approaches. Currently he uses dance as a therapeutic tool with individuals, couples and groups.

Naomi Aitchison remembers dancing alone, for the sheer joy of it, when she was four years old. Dancing was always what she wanted to do.

She has danced, studied dance and been a teacher of and lecturer in dance for many years. She was introduced to the work of Rudolf Laban in 1978 whilst undertaking training to be a secondary school drama teacher at Melbourne State College. This greatly influenced her own dance and her approach to teaching.

Since 1980 her endeavours have largely been directed towards recreational and therapeutic dance with elderly people in a wide range of settings. She was one of the first practitioners in Australia of dance with psychogeriatric and other disabled elderly populations. She regularly conducts in-service and other educational programs for students of dance, as well as carers of the elderly.

In 1986 she obtained the Graduate Diploma in Movement and Dance at the Institute of Early Childhood Development, Melbourne.

She is also a member of a group of dance therapy practitioners and students working towards the establishment of a dance therapy association in Australia.

Jenny Czulak has had a long career in educational broadcasting on radio and television with the Australian Broadcasting Corporation.

While in Britain on an Imperial Relations Trust scholarship in 1966, she took the opportunity of studying Peter Slade's body approach to drama. This fuelled further interest in expressive, creative dance movement on her return to Australia, in particular in the work of Johanna Exiner. Given the responsibility of creating a new weekly radio series of creative movement programs for the active participation of primary school students, Jenny, with guidance from Exiner and others, conceptualised, co-wrote and directed the successful "Free to Move!" programs which were broadcast by the ABC on a national basis for over three years.

She has done considerable movement work with sufferers from Alzheimer's disease; she conducts movement for well-being courses through the Council of Adult Education (Victoria, Australia) as well as "Moves You Can Make!"—a weekly movement and dance program for the isolated elderly, via conference phone.

Grad. Dip. Movement & Dance (University of Melbourne) 1979
Grad. Cert. Dance Therapy (University of Melbourne) 1988

Lisa Roberts—Diploma of Art, Victorian College of Art, Diploma of Education, Melbourne University, Graduate Diploma of Film & TV, Swinburne Institute.

Lisa is an exhibiting artist of drawings and computer animation, with a special interest in movement and dance. She studied creative movement with Johanna Exiner in the early eighties and as a result of this experience, taught drawing through movement. She storyboards and animates for film and television productions in Australia.

Her most recent project for exhibition is an interactive installation piece consisting of a 50's television with "wings" attached that randomly plays human gestures.

FOREWORD

Many influences are contributing to the evolution of dance therapy in Australia. Dance as a therapeutic mode has deep foundations in ancient health and healing ceremonies of the Aboriginal peoples who have inhabited the continent for at least 40,000 years. Ceremonial dance continues to play a part in Aboriginal health care. Australian dance therapists may wish to emulate new models of community health that incorporate traditional ritual practices with Western therapeutic technologies (Reid, 1984).

Dance therapy as an emergent professional field is being generated in an increasingly multi cultural Australia. As for the United States and other western countries, Australian dance therapy bears the lineage of 20th century Expressionism as reflected in European, American and Australian modern dance. *Dance Therapy Redefined* has origins in Johanna Exiner's early *Moderner Ausdruckstanz* training with Gertrud Bodenwieser in Vienna and is the first book on principles and practice of dance therapy in Australia.

I would like to establish a local context for *Dance Therapy Redefined*. By the early 1980s, the number of dance graduates working in therapeutic settings in the state of Victoria had grown into what was beginning to look like a professional community. Most practitioners had psychology, paramedical, special education, social work or nursing background in addition to a dance qualification; and such dual training continues to characterize career preparation for dance therapists. Australians have also benefited from intensive exposures to overseas specialists; notably Wynelle Delaney, Liljan Espenak and Dr. Marcia Leventhal.

The process of defining dance therapy in Australian terms entered a public stage in 1987 with the establishment of a Dance Therapy Working Party within the Victorian State Branch of the Australian Association for Dance Education. A comprehensive discourse was sought in order to establish a professional framework that would accommodate the range of populations, ethnic groups, practitioner backgrounds and demographic settings that may be involved in Australian dance therapy. After a year of deliberation, the following working definition was adopted:

> Dance therapy is based on the art and science of human movement. It offers movement experiences which, extending beyond the purely functional, engage both body and mind. Drawing on the therapeutic elements inherent in dance, therapists aim at restoring balance and integration in the areas of physical function, feelings and cognition.

Dance Therapy Redefined strengthens this Australian-grown conceptual framework. It provides a succinctly described model of dance therapeutic practice anchored in theories of body mind unity, in the aesthetic nature of dance, and in collaborative research. Autobiographical material from Johanna Exiner and Denis Kelynack enriches the presentation further. The book offers a departure from theoretical constructions that place dance therapy exclusively in the realm of psychotherapy; for example, the American Dance Therapy Association (1979) defines dance therapy as the "psychotherapeutic use of movement as a process which furthers the emotional and physical integration of the individual."

In *Dance Therapy Redefined*, the multi-sensory physicality of dance is the primary vehicle of therapy. Through what the authors term "reflection in motion," human beings may "dance further" into health. The aesthetic component, which may be realized through movement expression, that is "sensitive, mindful and imaginative," is seen as indispensable to the therapeutic process. Although words may be exchanged to question, reinforce, and conceptualize experience, it is *in the act of dancing* that therapy is realized. The role of therapist as teacher is affirmed. Clients are thus treated to the full promise of dance as a complete mode of learning.

I have enjoyed long and varied professional associations with all the authors of *Dance Therapy Redefined*, and I feel privileged to be writing this brief Foreword. The book constitutes a pioneering Australian contribution to the field of dance therapy, and will be welcomed by an increasing number of voices outside Australia that are calling for a return to dance as the central component of therapeutic practice.

Dr. Karen Bond
Senior Lecturer in Dance Education
The University of Melbourne

REFERENCES

AMERICAN DANCE THERAPY ASSOCIATION, "Definition of Dance Therapy," *American Journal of Dance Therapy,* 3(1), 1979.

REID, J. (ed.), *Body, Land and Spirit.* St. Lucia: University of Queensland Press, 1984.

PREFACE

Historically dance therapy has almost exclusively been defined as a form of psychotherapy. In our view, however, dance therapy is a discipline in its own right. Our method is anchored in our understanding of the structure and function of the human organism and the nature of dance.

We work with dance as the therapeutic material. Dance is the main vehicle of the therapy and it is in the act of dancing that the therapy is realised. Words are exchanged to question, to reinforce the process, to clarify and, where appropriate, to conceptualise what has been experienced.

This, we propose, is dance therapy in the truest sense.

As dance is the therapy and the instrument of dance is the body, it is the physicality of dance on which we focus. We do this by working towards physical changes as an integral part of change in the whole person.

It follows that because of the way we pay attention to the body, our approach is applicable to physical as well as psychical disturbances. We see the book as providing a platform from which others in dance therapy and related professions can take off, selecting, adapting and developing the material it contains for their specific purposes. While our text does not include individual case studies, the strategies we propose reflect the experience accumulated over many years of professional work. We have also taken account of the responses which groups of colleagues provided after participating in some of our introductory workshops. Their views contributed to the development and clarification of our thinking.

We believe the content of this book to be of value not only to those involved in the field of dance and dance therapy itself, but also to others with a more general interest in the function of dance in relation to the health and well-being of the community.

AUTHORS' NOTES

The authors have chosen to use, at times the female and at other times the male pronoun in preference to using either one consistently throughout.

The authors use the term *psychical* when referring to issues of the psyche and *psychological* when referring to psychology.

The authors use the term "client" (singular) interchangeably with "clients" (plural). However, examples given for work with a single client are in most instances applicable to group work.

ACKNOWLEDGMENTS

Johanna Exiner wishes to thank Dr. Gill Parmenter, Head of the School of Early Childhood Studies, University of Melbourne, for making available a private office to work in and access to office facilities; Pat Alsop, Senior Secretary in the General Office and Brenda Rush, Reader-Services Librarian, for years of advice and practical assistance and all staff members who contributed in one way or another to the completion of the manuscript; Dr. John Lloyd for his generous responses to repeated requests for information regarding the body/mind issue and Phyllis Lloyd for her consistent support and ongoing encouragement.

Johanna Exiner and Denis Kelynack express their gratitude to the Sidney Myer Fund (Melbourne) and its director, Michael Liffman, for a study grant to assist with the development of their work and to Mark Gordon, Executive Officer of the Australian Dance Council—Ausdance (Vic.) for administering the monies. Thanks to Norbert Hrouda whose expert videotaping formed an invaluable basis for examining the dance therapeutic process.

We both wish to put on record our recognition and appreciation of Naomi Aitchison's major contribution to the formulation and organisation of the text in all its aspects. We acknowledge with respect Jenny Czulak's constructive criticism, her focus on essentials and for giving so freely of her time in the preparation of numerous drafts. We are indebted to Lisa Roberts for the keen interest she took in our text which resulted in the book's dynamic illustrations. To Bob Exiner, who was always there when help was needed we say a very sincere personal thank you.

Finally we express our gratitude to Ingrid Barker for the great interest she took in our work, her patience in dealing with our many alterations and the care she took in preparing the final typescript; and to Karen de Ross who rescued us with a further typescript when Ingrid became unavailable.

INTRODUCTION—A PERSONAL ACCOUNT

The reason for offering an account of the direction I took from being a passionate dance student and performer to becoming at first a reluctant but finally a dedicated teacher, is its similarity to those taken by a number of dancers of my generation in the course of their professional life. For me, like for many others, the transition into dance therapy seemed to occur organically; I arrived, and I knew that was where I belonged.

I owe much to the cultural and professional environment in which this progression took place and gratefully acknowledge the many colleagues who encouraged and supported me. I only regret that in this brief history not all to whom thanks are due could be listed by name.

Johanna Exiner

I was introduced to dance in Vienna in Professor Gertrud Bodenwieser's children's classes.[1] At that time Bodenwieser was already Professor of Dance at the Academy for Music and the Performing Arts. Bodenwieser, a pioneer in what in Europe was given the name of *Moderner Ausdruckstanz* (Modern Expressive Dance) was hailed and respected as a liberator of dance, both in the topical and poignant themes she chose for her choreography as well as in her style, which she referred to as "expressionist". The work with us children was equally characteristic of her break away from the balletic tradition.[2]

I remained in Bodenwieser's children's classes until old and good enough to enter the Academy. I was fortunate in still being allowed to graduate in the third month of the Nazi regime in Austria, which had replaced Bodenwieser with a new director. Bodenwieser, who like myself, was of Jewish origin, had already fled to France. From there, and with the assistance of one of her most prominent group members still in Vienna,[3] a tour of Colombia was organised and again I was lucky, being accepted as a member. I did not regret abandoning my second year medical studies which I had undertaken as a second string to my bow concurrently with the Academy. I spent six wonderful months in South America dancing in Bodenwieser's gripping works on political, social and psychological themes. Equally inspiring was to perform her lyrical pieces as well as her charming Viennese flavoured sketches and, in contrast, her biting satires.

Whatever the content and however simply it might have been stated, Bodenwieser's choreography demanded complete involvement and, if danced as she conceived it, became a total experience. On reflection, I gradually realised that it was the *quality* of the dance arising from this experience which makes dance effective as therapy. The belief in dance I formed in my youth must have stayed with me subconsciously all along and has emerged as a guiding principle for the work we describe in this book.

In 1939 I moved from Colombia to Melbourne and started to teach.[4] From our base, the Studio of Creative Dance in which I joined Daisy Pirnitzer as co-director, we went out to give classes at a number of private girls' schools. At the Studio we conducted classes for children and adults, Shirley McKechnie being one of our distinguished pupils.[5] Daisy herself —we had studied dance together in Vienna from childhood onwards— was a highly imaginative teacher, choreographer and a powerful dancer.

At that time I did not enjoy teaching very much. I was young and wanted to dance. There was some scope for me to perform in dance recitals which we organised from the Studio. Occasionally we received invitations to dance at private functions and to contribute dance sections for plays and for opera.

In 1950 I took over the Studio and I was lucky. Many of the students who enrolled at that time, the late Margaret Lasica amongst them, were not only very gifted but also deeply committed to dance. Our style also attracted a number of talented men.

A very creative period began. Choreographing and performing were high priorities. The Modern Ballet Group was formed and I invited Margaret Lasica to co-direct it with me.[6] We presented regular seasons, mainly at Frank Thring's Arrow Theatre, but also at suburban and provincial centers. These were good times for me and my dance. I choreographed, I performed and did not worry so much about my teaching. And this relaxed attitude made the teaching ever so much more rewarding.

The work in schools eventually led to invitations by teacher training colleges to offer the then novel creative approach to dance. The first amongst them was the Kindergarten Training College (KTC),[7] and this became my professional and spiritual home.

KTC and Mercer House Teachers' College acquainted me with a developmental approach to education, influenced by Montessori, Bruner, Piaget and other such pioneers. Concurrently, I discovered Laban.[8] This resulted in a real breakthrough in my teaching. Young and old were introduced to Laban's elements of motion. Exploration became the main-stay of each class. Instead of making up movements and movement phrases, I provided students with guidelines for developing their own movement ideas and allowed form to grow organically from improvised material. I went overboard, to the extent that I neglected the teaching of skills, until I became aware how much skill contributes to creativity. On the positive side, I added an increased concern for individual progress to my curriculum-based approach.

Both of the teacher training colleges held the arts as a means of education in high esteem, and supported development in all the arts areas. At KTC I was given the opportunity to introduce creative dance for children to all students as a discipline in its own right, distinct from music to which it was traditionally linked. At the same time the study of dance was accepted as an elective major at undergraduate level. Due to the enlightened leadership of the College's Principal, Heather Lyon,[9] and her determined efforts, the next step was taken in 1977. This was to launch a Graduate Diploma of Movement and Dance, which I prepared with my close colleague Phyllis Lloyd.[10] The first of such degrees in Australia, its content reflected our commitment to dance in education, as well as our growing engagement in dance therapy.

1977 was an important year for dance in Victoria, not only because of the birth of the Graduate Diploma, but also because of the formation of the Australian Association for Dance Education (AADE),[11] which took off with flying colours. State branches were created and I became the first president of the Victorian Branch.[12] In the fifteen years of its existence it has actively promoted the educational aspects of dance in the widest possible sense. Sub-committees dealing with specific issues have been formed, prominent amongst them being the Dance Therapy Working Party which organised the first Australian Dance Therapy Conference in Melbourne in 1987, at which American dance therapist Dr Marcia B. Leventhal was the keynote speaker and main presenter. In 1992 the Working Party published *Dance Therapy Collections,* the first compilation of Australian dance therapy papers.

After my retirement from IECD in 1980, Karen Bond, another close colleague, initiated a Graduate Certificate in Dance Therapy, which I was asked to co-ordinate with her and in which we both taught.[13] The latest development in the rise of dance therapy in academe in Victoria has been the inclusion of Dance Therapy Studies at the Master of Education level.

My personal interest in dance therapy had been awakened quite early on: while naturally delighted with talented students I was attracted to strugglers and found it rewarding to help them over their physical and psychological hurdles. Psychology itself had quite a fascination for me ever since my student days in Vienna which at that time was buzzing with Freudian concepts. The subconscious, the Oedipus complex, hysteria etc., were discussed at home and in coffee lounges. Freudian slips were analysed at parties and entertained us for hours.

My first serious entry into psychology took place in Melbourne in 1950 when I began to work with one of the first fully trained Jungian psychologists in Australia. I continued this work for many years, experientially as well as through systematic private study. Later on I worked with a therapist who used a more eclectic approach and in doing so acquainted me with a number of recent developments in psychotherapy. Again I followed up personal experience with systematic reading of relevant sources. My interest in the function of the psyche never faded, but almost imperceptibly, my concern for the soma, the body, increased.

The challenge to apply what I had learnt was provided by a group of highly imaginative but equally dance-resistant art students at Mercer House in about 1973. To meet their needs I found myself moving back and forth between educational and therapeutic dance strategies. Working within a Laban-based framework enabled me to keep the borders fluid. I soon came to realise that fluid borders are a necessity for effectiveness in either field.

Putting my dance therapeutic efforts to the test, I invited Dr John Lloyd, psychiatrist, at the time in charge of the Therapeutic Community at Fawkner House, Mont Park Psychiatric Hospital, Melbourne, to observe and to give me his view on the therapeutic potential of the work I did with my art student group. His visit resulted in an invitation for me and Phyllis Lloyd to conduct regular dance therapy sessions at Fawkner House. There we further developed the therapeutic application of a Laban-based approach. The positive response we received from Fawkner

House led to work in other psychiatric institutions and to some consultations with clients who had physical problems.

In 1974 I undertook my first overseas study tour, supported by an Australia Council grant and generous study leave. In the UK I made the most of opportunities to refresh my understanding of the Laban approach and dance education in general. The visit to the USA which followed focussed on pure dance and on dance as therapy. Studying in the USA became an addiction and for the next decade I visited practically every two years, adding workshops in psychology to those connected with dance. This period provided enormous challenges to the thoughts and beliefs I had held, and gradually forced me to re-evaluate the work I had been doing in Australia.

I would have liked to have studied longer with Alwin Nikolais and Murray Louis,[14] to gain more insight and experience in the way they extended Laban concepts into highly technical as well as imaginative dimensions. The work of Erick Hawkins[15] had an even more profound influence on me. The humanity expressed in his style, demanding simplicity, humility as well as power, I found deeply moving. His philosophy and his view on people, society and art opened up new horizons of perception; so did the writings of the anthropologist Joseph Campbell, to which Hawkins drew my attention.[16]

My understanding of psychological issues was much enriched by participating in week-long intensives at the Centre for Studies of the Person, La Jolla, and at the Mental Research Institute (MRI), Palo Alto, California. At the former I had the good fortune to attend a session where the founder, Carl Rogers, demonstrated how he worked with a client. At the MRI I had the opportunity to meet and listen to the authors, Watzlawick, Weakland and Fisch, who had radically influenced my thinking through their book *Change* (1974), and I became acquainted with the views of other prominent members of the Institute.

The dance therapy workshop intensives at the University of California in Los Angeles and at the Naropa Institute in Boulder provided me with a wide range of information but often left me puzzled and in conflict. I soon discovered that the reason was that almost without exception dance was used as a way of "opening up" while the therapy itself occurred through verbal interpretation and analysis. The core of the therapy seemed to be psychology, not dance. The physicality of dance was not taken into account. Movement was not looked at in connection with the body, but only for what it expressed. Yet I *knew* that so much of myself and my needs as a person could not be separated from the body. Not to involve the body in the therapy caused me increasing frustration and made me realise that the approach to dance therapy I was pursuing had to move along a different path. Now my first priority was to acquire a better understanding of the relationship between body and mind.

When I began this research I was fairly comfortable to base my view on *interaction* of body and mind as propounded by Popper and Eccles in their book *The Self and Its Brain* (1977).[17] But the closer I came to establishing the body as a new basis for dance as therapy the more uneasy I grew with the thought of body and mind representing two separate entities. Was there a clear division between body and mind and if so, where was it? To justify a body approach to therapeutic dance, a clarification of that issue was essential. That was my quest over the last three years.

Observing people around me, family, friends, students, clients, and by no means least, myself, led me to the firm belief that the separation of body and mind was no longer tenable. What I saw, heard and felt pointed inevitably toward what some scientists refer to as psycho-physical monism, that is, a unified function of the human organism.

The evidence for monism, or systemic synchronism as other scientists referred to body-mind unity, gave me sufficient confidence to build a new approach to dance therapy on the conviction that we can reach the whole human organism through the body. Many of the insights gathered on the way remained partly submerged until my recent work with Denis, whose commitment to dance, to therapy and our partnership became a crucial factor in bringing them to the surface.

Our work together began towards the end of our final semester of teaching in the Graduate Certificate of Dance Therapy in 1989 when both Denis and I quite spontaneously expressed the wish to gain further knowledge and experience in each other's disciplines. We had no preconceived ideas as to how we would proceed. We allowed our working patterns to emerge gradually in the course of the first few sessions. Our roles, too, just established themselves: Denis began to dance. He became the "client" and I the "therapist." We both functioned as critical observers and commentators.

In the course of our practical work the importance of the body in the dance therapeutic process arose as the first of many distinctive features, all demanding further investigation. Gradually it became clear to us that the validity of our discoveries extended well beyond our particular pursuit and provided scope for a multiplicity of applications. To substantiate our findings and what could be deduced from them, we undertook extensive readings in a wide range of relevant literature, and tested what seemed important in our practical sessions.

In 1991 we applied to and subsequently received a grant from The Sidney Myer Fund[18] for the purpose of transcribing our audiotapes and the editing and some reconstruction of our videotapes. Both needed professional attention. Further work which had to be undertaken was to sift through records on dance and dance therapy, which I had gathered over a number of decades, and to select and categorise them for inclusion in our more recent findings.

In processing what had by now become a major project we realised that the material we were examining was substantial and deserved to be presented in book form. To do this would require more time and experience than either of us could contribute. We asked Naomi Aitchison and Jenny Czulak, both of whom had a considerable background in dance and therapy, if they would be interested in working with us. They not only agreed but became as convinced as we were that such a book would make an important contribution to the theory and practice of dance therapy.

Working together was challenging and productive; each of us bringing different talents to the quartet we had formed, the result of which is now before you.

NOTES

1. Gertrud Bodenwieser: Austrian dancer, teacher and choreographer, was born in Vienna in 1886 and died in Sydney, Australia in 1959. From Vienna she and her dance group toured Central Europe extensively and also visited Japan. After her tour through Colombia in 1938 she came to Sydney where she opened a school of modern dance and founded a new group which included Australian dancers. From Sydney, Bodenwieser and her group toured widely within Australia as well as visiting New Zealand, India and South Africa.

2. She introduced a liberated dynamic barre and floorwork in the style of Swedish gymnastics. "Centrework" she created newly for every class and it was practised with great variety in style and expression. Some of it became the topic for free improvisations, bringing each class to a delightful and profoundly rewarding closure. Improvised piano accompaniment was, on lucky days, provided by Marcel Lorber, Bodenwieser's dedicated pianist-composer and musical advisor. You could not but dance to his music.

3. Emmy Towsey who, like Bodenwieser, finally settled in Sydney. She established a school of creative dance for children and conducted adult classes. She was a major contributor to the Bodenwieser Archives founded and developed by Eric and Marie Cuckson in 1960.

4. I had done practice teaching in Vienna at the Bodenwieser school and shortly before Austria's *Anschluss* (unification) to the Third Reich, conducted women's classes in Rhythmic Gymnastics at a *Volkshochschule* i.e. a people's adult education centre.

5. Shirley McKechnie: after conducting her own School of Dance and contemporary dance company over the best part of seventeen years (from the mid fifties and early sixties respectively), became lecturer in dance at Rusden Teachers' College, Melbourne, where she introduced dance as a major within the Bachelor of Education course—a first in Australia. She was awarded an O.A.M. for her contributions to dance in 1987.

6. Margaret Lasica subsequently founded and directed the Modern Dance Ensemble in which great emphasis was placed on promoting the work of young dancers and choreographers. Within the last decade, her studio, Extensions, became the focal point for her teaching and for the advancement of contemporary dance exploration. Her sudden death in 1993 at the time when this text was being completed caused shock and distress to all who had known and worked with her.

7. In August 1973 the College was admitted as a constituent member of the State College of Victoria. It adopted the title: State College of Victoria—Institute of Early Childhood Development (SCV–IECD) and has since been amalgamated with the University of Melbourne and renamed the School of Early Childhood Studies, Institute of Education, University of Melbourne.

8. Rudolf Laban (1879–1958) Czech born dancer, choreographer, philosopher, educator and scholar. Best known for his identification of the principles of human movement and a system of movement observation and analysis which led to the development of *Labanotation*—the most widely used form of movement notation in the world. He established a method of movement education which blended with the philosophies of progressive educators such as J. Piaget, J.S. Bruner and Sir Herbert Read.

9. In 1992 Heather Lyon was awarded the degree of Doctor of Education *honoris causa* by the University of Melbourne.

10. Phyllis Lloyd is co-author of *Teaching Creative Movement* (1973) and *Learning Through Dance* (1987) and, in general, has always given my work invaluable support.

11. The founding members were Peggy van Praagh D.B.E., Shirley McKechnie O.A.M., Keith Bain O.A.M., Dr Warren Lett, Dr Peter Brinson (from the U.K.), Donna Greaves and myself. Renamed in 1992 Australian Dance Council (Ausdance) to cover an even wider range of dance activities.

12. The following statement, which I made at that time, I still believe to be valid for the dance community today and into the future.

> "Like everyone else, I have my preferences with regard to the many and diverse forms of dance which exist in society today. Yet, I respect them all

with one proviso and that is: I like them to be genuine, unadulterated and without trappings. I believe that any dance can fulfil its function by means of its own intrinsic strength and wealth of material, which we as teachers, choreographers and dancers must keep on exploring to the fullest extent. In working together we can ensure that:

• dance in schools and colleges will be educationally sound,
• as a leisure activity it will provide true recreation,
• in rehabilitation, its inherent and real therapeutic value will be tapped,
• in its role as a performing art it will evoke thought and feeling, open new vistas, refresh and entertain.

While many of us work from different platforms, we are linked through our love of and commitment to dance. How to make the most of our own and of each other's professional expertise in the service of the community, I personally see as one of the major aims of our association."

13. Karen Bond completed a Ph.D. entitled *"Dance For Children With Dual Sensory Impairments"* at LaTrobe University, Melbourne, in 1991—a first in the area of dance in Australia. Since then she has been responsible for the development and implementation of dance subjects leading to a Masters Degree in Education at the University of Melbourne.

14. Alwin Nikolais: Dancer, choreographer, director, teacher, composer (born 1912) created original costume and lighting effects and innovative music for dance. Murray Louis: Dancer, choreographer, teacher (born 1926) has been associated with Nikolais. Throughout his career danced in most of Nikolais' choreographies. They have separate dance companies but share a studio.

15. Erick Hawkins: Modern dancer and choreographer (born 1909). Danced with Balanchine and Ballet Caravan (a cooperative group) and for about ten years with Martha Graham. He formed his own company in the late 40s. His own works have always been primarily based on mythological themes.

16. Joseph Campbell (1904–1987), American anthropologist, philosopher, author and educator who particularly stressed the importance of myths in human existence. He pointed out the common ideas underlying the myths in cultures located in the most diverse parts of the globe.

17. *The Self and Its Brain: An Argument for Interactionism* was the result of the collaboration of Sir Karl Popper, philosopher, and Sir John Eccles, brain scientist.

18. The Sidney Myer Fund, based in Melbourne, was established in 1934 under the will of Sidney Myer. Its objectives are to provide funds for programs responding to community needs and for the development of new ideas.

CONTENTS

DANCE THERAPY REDEFINED

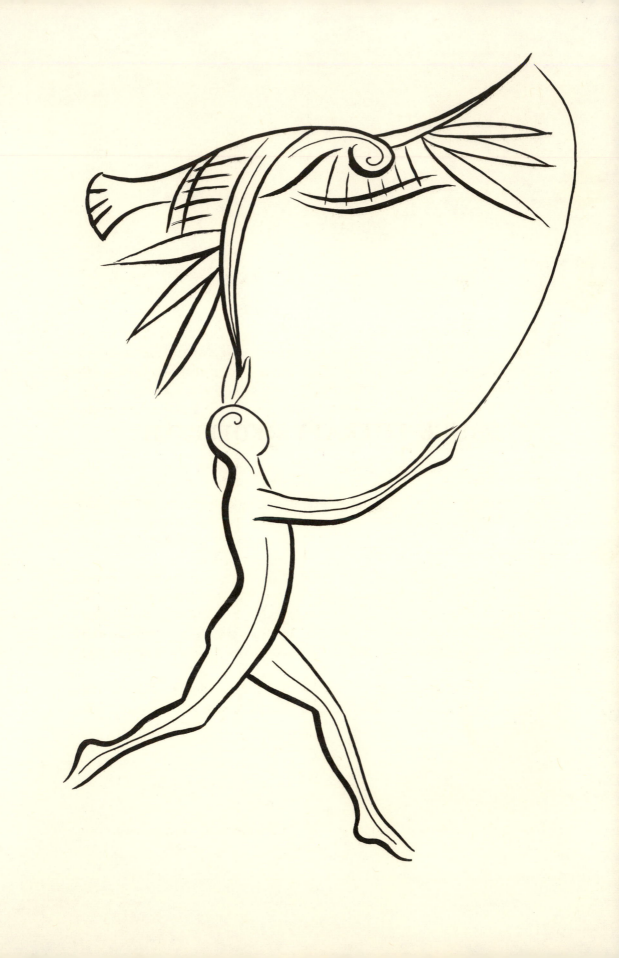

Chapter 1

THE BODY MIND ISSUE

"Man has no Body distinct from his Soul"
William Blake (1757–1827)

We have investigated the relationship between body and mind firstly because of its significance to the nature of health and sickness and secondly to establish the validity of taking a body approach to therapeutic dance. Because these terms, body and mind, are used somewhat differently by the various authors we shall be quoting, it needs to be clear that we accept that *mind* or *psyche* stands for the invisible, and *body* or *soma* for the visible aspect of the human organism.

In common with the authoritative sources we consulted we see the term *organism* as having no reductionist connotation. On the contrary, becoming better acquainted with the intricate functions of this thinking, feeling, moving, expressive being, has filled us with a true sense of wonder. The word *organism* encompasses our totality, our unity. Within ourselves we are finely differentiated yet we are whole.

We entered into our enquiry assuming that a state of closeness exists between body and mind which more often than not seemed to result in their functioning concurrently. We based this assumption on observations accumulated over many years living and working with people and directing our attention in particular to their attitudes to health and sickness.

Language often expresses the body-mind connection by showing the effects on the body of thoughts, events, relationships and feelings. For example:

"She makes me sick!"
"He's a pain in the neck."
"It gave me the shivers."
"I can't stomach this!"

Day-to-day behaviour is telling, too. In response to humour and joy,

3

shock and pain, people burst out laughing or crying, kick and scream, run and hug, with hardly a time span between the psychical cause and physical reaction. Where is the division between the physical and the mental in the involuntary trembling in fear, the upwardness of the body in moments of triumph, a person gagging when confronted with a gruesome sight? Being accident-prone is mostly linked with fatigue, yet at times seems the result of the subconscious wish to inflict injury on oneself.

A child is a striking example of unified functioning. Whether surprised, disappointed, curious, happy or sad, it seems that every cell in the body is affected by the experience. The response is total.

A distinctive body-mind connection is known to those of us actively involved in the arts. We, as dancers, know the experience of being in the dance "body and soul," sometimes only for a moment, but a moment remembered long afterwards for being other, unique, transcendent, a moment of wholeness.[1] Isadora Duncan is reported to have attained it in the simple act of sinking and rising which is said to have moved her audience to tears. Observing and experiencing such moments has very significant bearing on our concept of dance as therapy. So does listening to the quality of tone produced by a musician. When we describe his playing as "giving it his all," what do we mean? What is it that touches us so deeply? It is that the musician pours his inner experience into the physical act of music making through fingers, lips, and yes, the whole body: thus the music comes to life.

In the search for reference to the body-mind issue our attention was quite accidentally drawn to a book title: *The Seamless Web* by Stanley Burnshaw (1970). His first line immediately struck a chord: "Poetry begins with the body and ends with the body" (p. 1).

Later he quotes John Donne[2]: "To believe with John Donne that 'the body makes the minde'," he says "is to take into account everything that might affect the body: forces separate or in fusion, from without or from within, whose existence we have only started to recognise, whose nature and number may lie past our powers of perceiving." For this to be understood, Burnshaw comes to the conclusion that we should "learn our bodies and then from within look outward." In doing so, he continues "we come upon one finding with which all that may be discovered will have to accord: *the entire human organism always participates in any reaction*"
(p. 10).

Burnshaw (p. 12) describes the meaning of "such words as mind and emotion" by quoting René Dubos in *The American Scholar* (Spring 1965) who says: "They denote activities of the integrated organism responding as a whole to external or internal stimuli." He reinforces this with Dr. Kurt Goldstein's[3] statement: "We are always dealing with the activities of the whole organism the effect of which we refer at one time to something called mind and at another time to something called body" (pp. 13–14).

The physicist and philosopher of science, Mario Bunge,[4] to whose work we will refer in more detail later, says: "There is no harm in speaking of mental states or events provided we do not assign them to an immaterial, unchangeable and inscrutable entity but identify them instead with states and events of the brain" (1980, p. x). Bunge goes back in time to quote Charles Darwin who, in his notebooks, repeatedly stated his conviction that "The Mind is (a) function of (the) body" (p. 28).

Returning to Burnshaw: he refers to the poet Emily Dickinson who writes: "If I read a book and it makes my whole body so cold no fire can ever warm me, I know it is poetry. If I feel physically as if the top of my head were taken off, I know this is poetry." "Hence," he says, "everything we perceive and interpret by thinking processes become 'translated into organic processes' " (p. 15). We will look more thoroughly into the nature of this translation later on.

We conclude this first part of our body-mind discussion with the statement made by Pierce and Pierce, the authors of *Expressive Movement* (1989) which we quote in full, agreeing with Burnshaw that "paraphrase invites distortion" (p. 14). They say, "You are reading these words with your body, not just your eyes and your brain, but your whole body. The angle of your head, the depth of your breathing, the tension level of the muscles along your spine and around your mouth are parts of a pattern that is at this moment expressing your attitude and your response as you read. These so-called physical factors are not separate from your alertness, your receptivity, your capacity to focus, your sense of humour, the whole rich undifferentiated realm that you call 'reading' " (p. 14).

It was somewhat of a surprise to discover that Nietzsche[5] expressed a very strong and definite view on the body-mind issue in Zarathustra, I, 4, cited in R. J. Hollingdale (1973): "I am a body entirely" says Zarathustra "and nothing beside; and soul is only a word for something in the body." Nietzsche, says Hollingdale, saw psychology as a branch of physiology "with no distinct and circumscribed subject matter of its own" (p. 114). For Nietzsche "the object of study in psychology is increasingly not the condition of the 'psyche' but that of the whole organism" (p. 115).

Having arrived in philosophers' territory we found Joseph Campbell's answer to the body-mind question expressed in a manner most pertinent to our work: "The psyche is the inward aspect of the human body; it is the same the whole world over. The same organs, the same instincts, the same impulse system, the same conflicts, the same fears."[6]

Freud in one of his philosophical moods said [Rickman (ed.) 1953] "The ego is first and foremost a body-ego; it is not merely a surface entity but it is, in itself the projection of a surface . . . The ego is ultimately derived from bodily sensations, chiefly from those springing from the surface of the body. It may thus be regarded as a mental projection of the surface of the body" (p. 251).

Lowen (in Espenak, 1981) expands on this concept, making it even more relevant to our discussion of the body-mind connection: "The ego depends for its sense of identity upon the perception of the body. If the body is charged and responsive its pleasure function will be strong and meaningful and the ego will identify with the body. In this case the ego image will be 'grounded' in the body image. Where the body is 'unalive' pleasure becomes impossible and the ego disassociates itself from the body. The ego image becomes exaggerated to compensate for the inadequate body image" (p. 28).

From Freudian concepts we move to C. G. Jung, and in doing so we express our sincere appreciation to Martina Peter-Bolaender (1992) who, in her book *Tanz und Imagination* drew our attention to his view of the body-mind connection:

"As the human soul lives in inseparable unity with the body, psychology can only artificially separate itself from biological premises, and since the latter are valid not just for human beings but for the whole animate world, so they provide a certainty for a scientific base which surpasses that of psychological judgment which is only valid for the realm of consciousness."

And:

"Body and mind do not represent opposites but are the expression of one entity. The one is identical with the other, and doubt must be raised whether essentially the whole separation of mind and body is nothing else but a rationalisation conceived to facilitate comprehension, a distraction necessary for our understanding of one and the same reality from two perspectives which we have illegitimately endowed with independent existence" (p. 37).[7]

Rollo May (1969) looks at body-mind from a different, rather more practical perspective: "My body is an expression par excellence of the fact that I am an individual. Since I am a body separate from others as an individual entity, I cannot escape putting myself on the line some way or other—or refusing to put myself on the line, which is the same issue." And further: "The fact that my body is an entity in space, has this motility and this particular relation to space which my movements give it, makes it a living symbol of the fact that I cannot escape in some way or other 'taking a stand'." As May points out: "we say someone is 'upright,' 'straight,' or the opposite, 'cringing,' 'ducking,' all referring to will and decision as shown through the position of the body" (p. 240).

"Even more interesting," he says, "is the body as *language* of intentionality.[8] It not only expresses intentionality; it *communicates* it." "Obviously it" (the language of the body) "communicates much more than the bright intellectualized talking of the sophisticated patient who chatters for months in order to avoid awareness of his own underlying feelings" (p. 241). Here, May points directly at those aspects which show people's resistance to accepting the body as an integral part of their being.

It becomes abundantly clear that, even in the attempt to prevent the body from "speaking" one is saying something about it. People may believe that they can hide their thoughts, saying only what they want others to hear, yet body language often contradicts verbal expression.

Robin Williams of the ABC Science Show put it bluntly: "So much of your personality is being flesh."[9]

[In many instances the body does *not*, of course, represent the outer aspect of the psyche, such as in the case of persons suffering from genetic malformation or where sickness or accidents have caused lasting damage to their bodies.]

Enlightening and convincing because of the power with which they are made are Eric Berne's views in *Beyond Games and Scripts* (1976). In his opinion the growing child is fitted out with a *script* created by the values and the behaviour of parents and other carers, including grandparents. Scripts can be productive or destructive, but Berne says, "the script is a way to structure the time between the first Hello at mother's breast and the last Goodby at the grave" (p. 225).

He addresses himself to the issue of scripts in relation to personality problems: "For each patient there is a characteristic posture, gesture, mannerism, tic, or symptom which signifies that he is living 'in his script' or has 'gone into' his script. As long as such 'script signals' occur, the patient is not cured, no matter how much 'progress' he has made. He may be less miserable, or happier, living in his script world, but he is still in that world and not in the real world, and this will be confirmed by his dreams, his outside experiences, and his attitude toward the thera-pist . . . " (p. 278).

So far, all our observations and the study of sources confirmed our belief that body and mind form an entity. But belief, we felt, was not enough. We had to address the critical questions: How is the human organism constructed for unified functioning? How does the "script" become ingrained in the body? By what means does the "script" affect bones and muscles? What are the channels through which feelings, of love, for people, for music, for life itself, as well as feelings of despondency, frustration, sorrow, reach "the flesh"?

And conversely: *how does working through the body in dance reach the whole person?* How does it loosen ingrained patterns? How does it improve or restore the smooth functioning of the organism, as it so obviously does?

Mario Bunge who deals with these questions extensively and in consid-erable depth points out in the introduction to his work, *The Mind Body Problem* (1980), that even addressing the issue is hindered by a tacit acceptance of "psychophysical dualism," namely, the doctrine that mind and body are separate entities. "Only very recently," he says, "have scientific research programs focussed on the issue, still hampered though by the traditional metaphysical approach to the question it begs" (p. xiv).

He divides those who deal in some depth with the body-mind issue into two categories:

1. psychophysical dualists who "are united in the conviction that the mind has an existence apart from the brain" (p. 2), and
2. psychophysical monists who "hope to be able to understand the mental by studying the brain components and their interactions" (p. 2).

Bunge is a psychophysical monist and with him we believe that the interaction does not occur between a non-material metaphysical mind and a material body but that "The so-called psychophysical (or psycho-somatic) relations are interactions of the subsystems of the brain or between some of them and other components of the organism" (p. 21). For instance, Bunge says: "The coupling between the CNS* and the

---

*Central Nervous System

endocrine glands . . . is so intimate that, although the two can be distinguished anatomically, they cannot be separated physiologically. Neural systems activate endocrine organs via blood-borne hormones. In turn, hormonal signals activate neural systems . . . " (p. 37).
And later: "disturbances of nonmental (e.g. metabolical) bio-functions may influence mental states and, conversely mental events, such as acts of will, may influence nonmental bodily states" (p. 84).

Bunge calls the philosophy he develops "emergentist materialism"[10] and claims that it "is the only *philosophy* [italics added] that enjoys the support of all the sciences" (p. 219). In the field of medical practice however, we find that the case of body-mind relation is treated with great reservation: "Clinical signs, symptoms and syndromes which clearly signal interaction between somatic dysfunction and the mental process have too often been left aside, untouched by necessary interdisciplinary discussion, education, critical review and research." So say Öhman et al, editors of *Interaction Between Mental and Physical Illness* (1989, p. vii).[11] They also consider that: "Psychosomatic states in the form of somatization of anxiety, aggression and sexuality, chronic pain syndromes, sleep disorders, and gastrointestinal, dermatological, or gynaecological problems, illustrate where medical professional interest has been insufficient or absent. Many of these problems have been left to paramedical or even lay intervention. The present wave of 'alternative' medicine (psychologically and somatically orientated) may in fact be to a large extent a logical consequence of neglect by both the medical profession and the public health system. The public need for understanding and acceptance of body-mind interaction has not been adequately evaluated." (p. vii)

The kind of "interaction" which is referred to here does *not* deal with that of a nonmaterial, metaphysical mind and a material body but with interactions between the various systems within the "material" organism. Perhaps it is important to note here that none of our sources denigrate what we call mind, but rather raise the status of *matter* in all its myriad forms.

Continuing our investigations into psychosomatics we find Wolman, the author of *Psychosomatic Disorders* (1988),[12] expressing the opinion that looking at the organism through a psychosomatic lens gives us a more realistic picture of the roots of health and illness. Wolman says: "Psychosomatic and somatopsychic phenomena are daily occurrences. Emotions affect the circulatory and gastrointestinal systems and an intake of food and liquid affects mental functions. In certain instances psychological

factors affect physical health and do damage to the human body"
(p. 48).

In *Psychoneuroendocrinology,* Vol. 14, 1989, David Saphier expands on
this concept: "For many years, the central nervous system and the immune
system were considered as entirely separate entities in terms of maintenance of the state of well-being of the organism. However, it also has
been understood for some time that psychological factors, such as stress,
e.g. following bereavement, may lead to decreased immunocompetence
and increased incidence of disease" (p. 63). He also states that: "Putative
mechanisms . . . exist by which the immune system may 'talk' to the
nervous system" (p. 65).

The idea though "that psychological states can affect the outcome of
human disease is an old one," says A. J. Dunn (1989). "The Greek author
Galen wrote around 200 AD that melancholy women are more suscep-
tible to breast cancer than sanguine women" (p. 251).* In 1990 Dunn
wrote: "recent reports have begun to substantiate some of the fundamental beliefs in psychoneuroimmunology, such as the concept that psychological state has important impact on immunocompetence. There is also
growing evidence that immune function can have an important impact
on the psychological state" (p. 103). Hence, as Enrico Camara (1989)
points out: "it is important for all biopsychologically oriented physicians
to understand the network that connects the central nervous system and
the immune system" (p. 140).

Despite the caution exhibited in the medical profession our observations and research reveal an increasing number of medical practitioners
do accept the psychosomatic nature of many illnesses. Increasingly,
attention shifts from the identified symptom to the state of the whole
organism. General acknowledgment of synchronous function of the organism at all times may not be too far off.

NOTES

1. It is interesting to note that "healing" is derived from the word "whole." The
   verb "to heal" therefore means to become whole again.
2. English poet, 1572–1631.
3. Author of *The Organism,* Boston Beacon Press 1963.
4. Mario Bunge is Head of the Foundation and Philosophy of Science Unit at

---

*Even earlier, in 400 B.C., Aristotle argued that a change in the soul produced a change in the shape of
the body and vice versa.

McGill University, Montreal. He was born in the Argentine, is a Ph.D. in physics and was formerly Professor of Physics and Experimental Physics at the University of Buenos Aires and Professor of Philosophy at the University of La Plata.

5. Friedrich Nietzsche (1844–1900), German philosopher, wanted to replace the alleged Christian doctrines of weak, ascetic and submissive behaviour with the "will to power" of a select number of "supermen" who can control themselves and are superior to the rest of humanity. He believed dance to be a basic artistic activity expressing human attitude to life.

6. Quote from the series *The Power of Myth* shown on ABV2 (Australian National Television channel) Oct. 1991. A production of Apostrophe S. Productions Inc., Alvin H. Perlmutter, Inc., Public Affairs Television Inc. U.S.A. 1988.

7. Translated by the authors, the excerpts are taken from C. G. Jung *Gesammelte Werke,* vol. 8: *Die Dynamik des Unbewußten,* Zurich 1971, pp. 133 and 370.

8. Rollo May defines the term intentionality in this way:

    "Intentionality is what underlies both conscious and unconscious intentions. It refers to a state of being and involves to a greater or lesser degree the *totality* of the person's orientation to the world at that time" (p. 234).

9. Radio interview with Doug Aiton, 24.9.92, Australian Broadcasting Corporation.

10. According to Bunge there are three types of materialism:

    1. *Eliminative Materialism* which holds that there is no such thing as mental, everything is material-physical. There is no mind-body problem as there is no mind.

    2. *Reductive Materialism* which holds that the C.N.S., as a physical entity, differs from other physical systems *only* in complexity. The brain is *nothing* but an aggregate of cells, if we understand the cells we understand the mind.

    3. *Emergentist Materialism* holds that the mind is a set of emergent bioactivities. This allows for the specificity of the mental without accepting a duality of body and mind. Mental states are a subset of brain states. Mental states, events, and processes emerge relative to those of the cellular components of the brain. Bunge (pp. 5–6, 8, 21)

11. R. Öhman, H. L. Freeman, A. Franck Holmkvist and S. Nielzén were the editors of *Interaction Between Mental and Physical Illness* which contains the proceedings of the fifth workshop on that subject set up by a special study group of the European Medical Research Councils (EMRC) in 1987. Formed in 1971 EMRC became a Standing Committee of the European Science Foundation. Its stated aims were the initiation and stimulation of international cooperation in biomedical research.

12. Wolman describes this publication, in the preface, as:

    "an encyclopaedic book on psychosomatic disorders written for neurologists, psychiatrists, psychologists, psychiatric social workers and other mental and physical health professionals."

Plenum Medical Book Co. N.Y., London 1988.

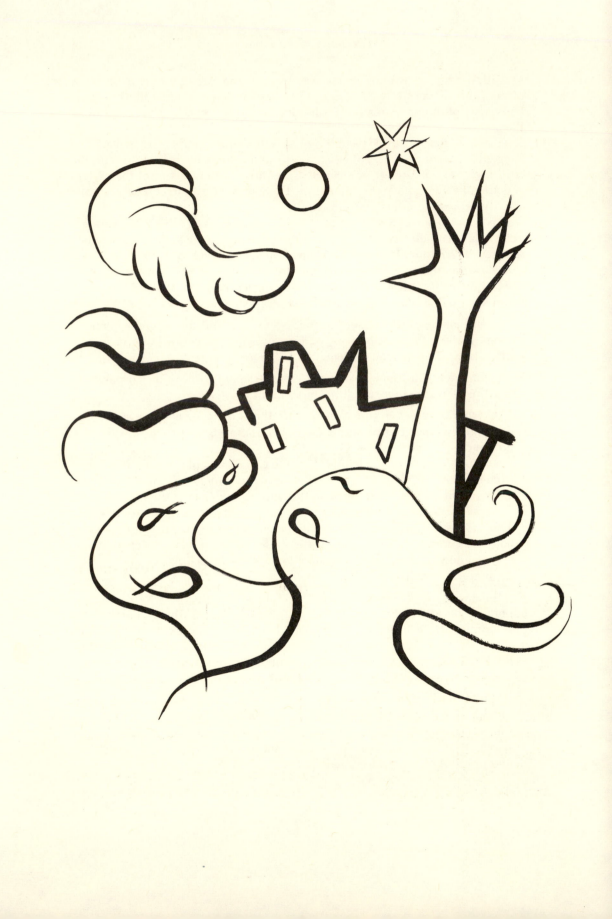

Chapter 2

DANCE AND AESTHETICS IN
THE CONTEXT OF DANCE THERAPY

"... aesthetic perception is not something rare and exotic, unless life is so lived that it comes to be considered unnatural. What could be more natural than simply to look out upon the world and take interest in its sights and sounds, its movement and expressiveness."
Stolnitz, J. *Aesthetics and the Philosophy of Art Criticism,* 1960, p. 44.

Since dance is our chosen therapeutic material it is imperative to ask what is its essential nature? What is this thing called dance?

Even Roderyk Lange, in his book *The Nature of Dance* (1975), offers only a number of definitions, yet none are totally satisfying. It seems that one can talk *about* dance, one can describe particular dances, but dance itself, like music, is difficult to capture in words.

Much has been written about the different forms in which dance manifests itself. Howard Gardner (1983) provides a dynamic study of its purposes: "Dance," he says, "can reflect and validate social organization. It can serve as a vehicle of secular or religious expression; as a social diversion or recreational activity; as a psychological outlet and release; as a statement of aesthetic values or an aesthetic value in itself." Dance can teach, it can be liturgical, and it can reflect on tribal rituals such as initiation. It can serve to placate the elements, it can invoke supernatural powers. It can be the instrument for sexual selection. Dance can symbolise the important events of a community or celebrate its traditional work patterns, such as sowing and reaping. And it can include, as Gardner says, "several of these functions, either simultaneously, at different times, or in different milieux" (p. 223). The diversity of dance forms is staggering, but not surprising if we take into account the different cultures from which dance grew, and the multifarious purposes it can address. Adding to this diversity are the vast numbers of artists who developed their own personal styles.

What is important for us in Gardner's work is that he speaks about dance "providing a psychological outlet and release," which we assume

13

he considers to be therapeutic. And his comment on dance having an "aesthetic value in itself" merits appreciation since dance for dance's sake, for simply savouring the experience of the movement, is not often acknowledged. The symbolic nature of dance in the various other purposes he identifies is more commonly understood.

Dance is an ancient art. It happens because we humans are born with the faculty of dancing. It is a form of human behaviour which only needs a favourable environment to be cultivated and developed.

But are we coming any closer to what this thing called dance really is? Some may even doubt that attributes common to all dance exist, yet we will propose that they do. To begin with there is something that connects all dance and that, of course, is the body.

The body is the instrument of dance and an extremely versatile one. Choreographers such as Martha Graham, Pina Bausch, Mats Ek and Paul Taylor have required dancers to use their bodies in ways one would have thought physically impossible. Yet no matter what astonishing acrobatic feats are performed (nor what minimal gestures made), there exists for the dancer and for the viewer a shared awareness of essential criteria without which dance remains merely movement.

One criterion is the dancer's (the doer's) identification with motion, during which, in Linda Leah's* words, "you are inside the movement with all your faculties." In giving over to the movement, "body and soul," the dancer becomes one with it, and this kinetic identification also applies to the viewer. The American writer and dance critic, John Martin (1965), describes the viewer's response as "inner mimicry" (p. 55),[1] an attribute which the dance critic requires in order to understand a performer, the teacher to educate a student, and the therapist to work with a client.

The world-famous choreographer, dancer and teacher, Murray Louis (1973) defines the essence of dancing as "sensing the nature of movement."[2]

Laban† places major emphasis on dance action needing to arise from within. The German word Laban employed was *Antrieb* which, in the English version, became "effort." It seems to us that "impulse" would have described the meaning of *Antrieb* much better. Laban believed that this impulse must come from the center. It is the center which sustains the movement thus released, even if it is no more than flicking a finger.

---

*Dance educator, Melbourne, Australia

†See Preface, Note 8, p. 9.

Such "centered" movement contrasts with that described as "peripheral." Peripheral movement gives out a different message. We are not referring here to those peripheral movements which are intentional, such as in a dance of "being casual," but to non-centered movement which may reflect a lack of depth or an unconnectedness on the part of the dancer.

The question arises, where and what is this center? In Ancient Greece it was thought to be located in the diaphragm and was considered the seat of the soul. Isadora Duncan adopted this idea and embellished it, talking of a central inner switch she needed to turn on in order to release herself into dance.

Dance, created or recreated, will only live if, as Franzisca Boas (1971) puts it: "a transformation takes place within the person, a transformation which takes him out of the ordinary world and places him in a world of heightened sensitivity." This she says "is the source of dance as contrasted with movement" (pp. 21, 22). Barbara Mettler (undated) expresses herself similarly. If, for instance, in walking she is merely concerned with where to go and how to get there, then she says "the utilitarian aspect of the movement dominates my experience and it is just an ordinary walk." If, on the other hand, she becomes engrossed in the movement for its own sake "its purposeful stride, its lively swing, its steady beat, its constant forward direction—then, in that moment, dominated by the feeling of the movement," she says, "I am dancing" (p. 7).

It seems then that *this thing called dance* depends on the dancer, a concept lyrically expressed by W.B. Yeats:[3]

> "O body swayed to music, O brightening glance
> *How can we know the dancer from the dance?*" [italics added]

We believe that this unification of dancer and dance occurs when movement is carried out with *sensitivity, mindfulness and imagination.* And there is something further. Boas speaks of "transformation," Mettler of being "dominated by the feeling of the movement." What they are describing in different words is a change, an entry into another dimension of experience. A new way of knowing is encountered. We have entered the *dance mode* which transports us into the domain of aesthetics. What this entry feels like, some describe as the "eureka" experience. Arthur Koestler (1964) refers to it as an "oceanic" feeling (p. 88).[4] It elates, expands, excites and fulfills.

Let us now investigate the concept of aesthetics as we understand and use it. The word itself comes from the Greek: *aisthanomai* "to perceive".

Its original meaning refers to sense perception as opposed to intellectual processing and only became a term to describe the quality of beauty around the eighteenth century. In this book we use "aesthetics" in its original meaning; aesthetic perception enables us to experience and appraise the environment through the senses without primarily involving the intellect; for instance, one may be attracted or repelled by the tone of a speaking voice regardless of the message it conveys. Today aesthetics are often confused with a sense of style, but style in our opinion represents the "character" artists give to their work. Examples of dance *styles* would be Balanchine's flowing and intertwining group patterns, Graham's contractions, turned up toes and cupped hands or Humphrey's "fall and recovery."

The biological root for the aesthetic, the "sensuous" experience in dance, is the *kinesthetic* sense, about which Telford and Sawrey (1968) make the following comment: "The kinesthetic sense endings are located in the muscle-spindles, the tendons and the joint surfaces." Furthermore, they point out that "every muscular contraction and every tension change in a muscle is not only a response but also serves as a stimulus" (p. 118). Oliver Sacks (1986) talks of "this vital 'sixth sense' by which the body knows itself, judges with perfect, automatic, instantaneous precision the position and motion of all its moveable parts, their relation to one another, their alignment in space" (p. 46).

And he also states: "One may be said to 'own' or 'possess' one's body — at least its limbs and moveable parts — by virtue of a constant flow of incoming information, arising ceaselessly, throughout life, from the muscles, joints and tendons. One has oneself, one IS oneself, because the body knows itself, confirms itself, at all times, by this sixth sense. I wondered how much the absurd dualism of philosophy since Descartes might have been avoided by a proper understanding of 'proprioception' " (pp. 46, 47).*

H. Rieder, in the German journal *Tanzen* (3.89) offers as synonyms for the kinesthetic sense: muscle awareness (*Muskelsinn*), energy awareness (*Kraftsinn*), sense of motion (*Bewegungsgefühl*), sensitivity (*Sensibilität*), body awareness (*Körperempfindung*), perception of motion (*Bewegungs-empfindung*),† with the comment that some of these are subject to controversy (p. 21).

---

*For further information on proprioception, see Appendix 1.

†Authors' translations.

In dance a fusion occurs between the purely physical (we call it quantitative) measurable aspect of kinesthesia, and its qualitative, immeasurable companion. This fusion provides the person dancing not only with the knowledge of where he is in time and space, which parts of his body he energizes and how he coordinates movement; it also, and most importantly, enables him to experience the aesthetic quality of motion itself, to *taste* the intrinsic nature of a leap, a fall, an abrupt change of direction, an acceleration, a slowing down, and in very special contrast to movement, moments of stillness.

"To know movement," says Margaret H'Doubler (1966), "one must attend to *the sensations of his own moving body* [italics added] thereby discovering movement to be a highly stimulating experience whose sensations can be held in consciousness *where they can be recognized, compared, evaluated and where ideas can be formed about them*" [italics added] (p. xxi). H'Doubler refers to this experience as aesthetic "feedback" (p. xxv).

This leads us to the highly significant issue, namely that of *reflection in motion.*

Reflection in motion rather than in words, is central to the dance therapy we propose. And by *dancing further* about what has been discovered in the initial exploration, more can be extracted and learned from it. Reflection can take place even if the dancing is restricted to very simple movements. It enables recapitulation, the discarding of what is irrelevant, retaining what is valuable and developing it further. This is the dance equivalent of clients in verbal therapy, checking the validity of what they are saying, expressing themselves unambiguously, and learning to understand better what they have discovered. It is the dancing which will tell how to proceed and what choices to make.

All arts make demands on the body but dance does so totally. The dancer needs to bring to it all of himself, his whole personality, *which includes the body.* Failure to address the body in the dance therapy process would therefore deny the client the benefits of the physicality of dance. What is more, the demand which dancing makes on all facets of the human organism gives it the power to provide *integration* within the person. Integration is widely recognised as one of the major aims of any therapy. In dance, integration takes place in the domain of aesthetics.

In dance therapy we have encountered it on occasions never to be forgotten, such as when in a dance therapeutic group, a painfully withdrawn chronic schizophrenic was encouraged to extend his arm upwards.

After initial assistance, the arm seemed to start travelling of its own accord, not far, just a little further than the man's head. Yet he said with his face alight: "I can't remember ever having reached that far!" In another therapeutic group was a young drug addict. At the end of a passionate improvisation he flung himself onto his knees, opened his arms, and throwing back his body exclaimed: "This feels as good as a fix!" Both men had felt movement way beyond the purely functional. Both had experienced a transformation, they had entered the aesthetic dimension.

It is our view that the aesthetic experience is accessible as much to the handicapped as to budding ballerinas. There is no doubt in our minds that even with minimal movement a transforming dance experience is possible, and that in this transformation lies one of dance's powerful therapeutic effects.

Regarding the question of how dance can be therapeutic for the physically handicapped, our observations show that the energy produced in the healthy, undamaged parts of the body can be experienced as a *resonance* throughout the organism and can unexpectedly trigger off responses. In other words every cell in the body has the potential to participate.

Therapeutic dance with any population or in any situation incorporates thinking, feeling and willing. Movements do not become less authentic when monitored by the intellect. We believe it to be unnatural to cut out the thinking process, the supreme attribute evolution has endowed us with. If we use our intellects for observing, for selecting, for organizing and for making choices then they become "competent servants rather than incompetent masters" (Gelb 1987, p. 34).

We need to "think-feel" as Hawkins[5] says, and use our will without allowing dominance of one over the other, except when we choose to do so.

In dance as therapy, however, we suspend the critic and the analyst in ourselves, yet may still wish to pay attention to what we do. It seems erroneous to believe that feeling and thinking are engaged in a fundamental conflict. On the contrary, they enhance and reinforce each other.

In conclusion, we believe there is no therapeutic dance as such, just as there is no "special" dance for children, or for the aged; dance becomes educational or therapeutic in the hands of specialists. While adapting dance to the needs of their respective populations, therapists and teachers ensure that the essential nature of dance stays intact.

NOTES

1. John Martin (1965) also states, "when . . . functioning not as a dancer but as a spectator his experience of movement . . . will give him an increased responsiveness through the channel of inner mimicry" (p. 298).
2. Murray Louis from the commentary to the film "Motion," the fifth in his series *Dance as an Artform*, Chimera Productions, New York 1973.
3. From "Among Schoolchildren viii."
4. Sigmund Freud, in "Civilization and its Discontents" Standard Works, Volume xxi, The Hogarth Press and The Institute of Psychoanalysis, London (p. 64) attributes the term to Romain Rolland who used it in a letter to Freud describing it as a term for eternity and limitlessness.
5. Statement made in class by Erick Hawkins in 1981.

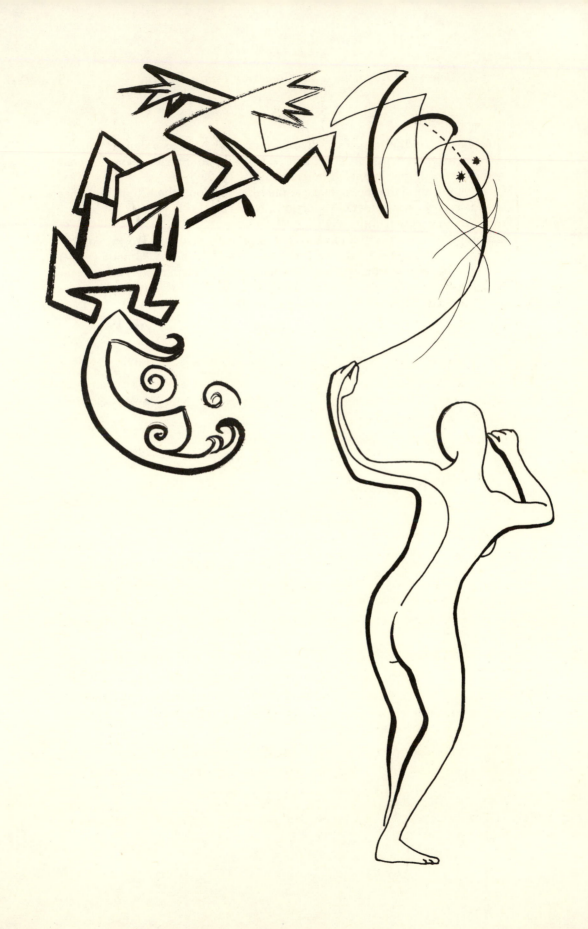

Chapter 3

THE CONCEPTUAL FRAMEWORK

"Beware that you do not lose the substance by grasping at the shadows."
Aesop's Fables: The Dog and the Shadow.

I. THE DANCE THERAPEUTIC PATH

We see the nature of the dance therapy process as a journey along the therapeutic path, a journey which remains open-ended. Along this path as much is learnt from the hurdles that are met, the detours taken, as when the way is clear.

Overall the journey has five phases:

- ENTRY
- EXPLORATION
- CORE ACTION
- REVIEW, and
- CONCLUSION.

ENTRY establishes the preparedness of the client to become acquainted with dance as the therapeutic medium. This can be immediate or a gradual process over a number of sessions, during which time a commitment will develop, or else a decision will be made to seek alternative therapy.

EXPLORATION, by means of improvisation (DEDUCTIVE APPROACH), or guided movement experiments (INDUCTIVE APPROACH), uncovers the links in the chain of circumstances which led to the client's current condition, be it a physical complaint, a psychical disturbance or both.

A wide focus is required for the exploratory phase. This focus will be narrowed down and centered on the emerging *themes** that call for

---

*A theme within the context of the therapeutic path, as well as in that of a session, represents distinctive movement configurations, dance motifs or qualities of motion which specifically deal with the physical or psychical symptom.

21

attention. These themes will become the substance of the next phase which we call CORE ACTION.*

In CORE ACTION the work becomes specific in the sense that we select relevant movement material from the themes, then develop and clarify it. In the course of this, *recognition* grows of the nature of the clients' problem and the kind of actions to be taken. Over a period the work gains in depth via shifts in body-mind functioning, manifested in changes of posture and manner of movement, and in attitudes to everyday life. However, these changes will be transitory unless they are reinforced and gradually integrated, through further work in sessions, by practising at home, and in applying subsequent resolutions to daily living.

REVIEW is a transitional phase where the dance experiences and their relevance to daily living are reflected on and refined. Often additional insights will be gained at this time and previous resolutions reinforced.

CONCLUSION is the act of stepping away from the therapy. Clients have reached a point at which they feel confident of managing their lives in a more satisfactory and productive manner, both physically and psychically; when the issues of day-to-day living are no longer overshadowed by therapeutic concerns, and they feel that what has been learnt will be retained and that understanding will continue to grow.

II. MODEL OF A SESSION

The model for each session is a micro-version of the therapeutic path.

In individual or in group work we feel our way into what kind of movement quality is needed for ENTRY, whether to stimulate or pacify, or whether to accept that clients may wish to talk about what has happened for them since the previous session. The ENTRY phase always includes *sensitising,* tuning up and preparing the body for action.

This leads naturally into EXPLORATION, where movements which have arisen during the entry phase will now be experimented with. Then a selection is made of those which seem to be physically beneficial or emotionally significant, and they become the theme for CORE ACTION.

---

*Themes demanding CORE ACTION do not only emerge during EXPLORATION. They may appear unannounced at any time.

For example, during EXPLORATION we may have observed a rigid *posture,* or a dominant movement *mode,* both of which are limiting, and hence part of the client's problem, requiring modification or change. The measures chosen in response would offer gradual release for the rigidity or in the case of a limiting movement mode experimentation with alternatives.

In CORE ACTION thematic material will be taken through a process of *development.* Tactics such as changes in tempo, pathways and energy, repetition, variations and further movement discoveries, may be introduced. Clients may go off on tangents or detours which may indicate the need for additional goals. Some may choose alternatives to this development, letting go of the initial theme and returning to exploration. The patterns which have emerged during the development will become more informative and effective through *clarification.*

This means movement will be refined by more careful attention to its psycho-physical content and the way it is put into action. *Recognition* of further therapeutic steps to be taken will also be gained in the course of the CORE ACTION.

REVIEW is a time for reflection in dance or words or both. We look at the material which has come up in the previous stages then, together with clients, we decide what would be valuable for them to take away and work on. This could consist of further work in dance and also a course of action to try in everyday life.

Sessions are best rounded off with a CONCLUSION in the form of a dance even if it does not flow on from the preceding work. It is important not to step out of the arena of dance too suddenly, rather to feel one's way to an ending, allowing time for a sense of completion to occur, and staying with that for some moments. A convention can be established by agreement in advance, that the client indicates readiness to conclude the dance for instance by an extended stillness followed by a deep breath. Home practice would not be suggested to clients preferring to stay with the thoughts and feelings that have emerged from the CORE ACTION, wishing to let them "simmer". This is really reviewing in a free-flow manner. REVIEW and CONCLUSION run into each other here.

Along the path we, as therapists, are mindful of the importance of remaining flexible, of the need not to adhere rigidly to the phases we have described. No two human beings fall into one identical mould, neither do circumstances nor situations. This proviso applies equally to the models described for the therapeutic path as it does to individual sessions.

III. GOALS

The overall goal of our therapeutic work is the restoration of psycho-physical health or learning to cope adequately with an unalterable state. In cases of very severe impairment often no more than a temporary relief can be achieved.[1]

We differentiate, as probably most therapists do, between long- and short-term goals. A long-term goal could be seen as a thread which indicates the general direction the therapy is likely to take. Rather than being obvious at the start this thread may only be identified along the way. Short-term goals are pursued in response to the more obvious symptoms or issues which clients present (initially or in the course of the therapy) and which require to be relieved by immediate attention.

IV. FUNDAMENTAL PRINCIPLES

Our method rests on a number of fundamental principles. We discuss each in isolation, fully aware that in practice they overlap and interweave. None are mutually exclusive. Our approach is based on developmental precepts and is consequently client-centered; the needs of clients determine where to start and how to proceed. The way we work towards achieving therapeutic goals is to bring about change.

The questions which immediately arise are:

change   What brings about change and what obstructs it?
How do we recognize it?
How do we know it is appropriate?

We hold the view that change is brought about by a process of learning.[2]

learning   Given that our therapeutic material is dance and dance takes place in the *body* so must the learning. As it is dance through which we learn, and dance engages the whole person so must the learning. All true learning (which is more than acquiring information and skills) generates change. Dance provides true learning in the fullest sense.

Our working method has some aspects in common with the body therapies, in particular with the Alexander Technique as described by Michael Gelb in his book, *Body Learning* (1987). However we do not stop with the body. We take the body learning into sensitive, mindful and imaginative movement, that is dance, with the certainty that it will act upon the whole organism.

unlearning   Learning, in the dance therapeutic sense, will be preceded by unlearning of fixed and unproductive attitudes, actions and ways of moving. As F. Mathias Alexander[3] says: "You can't do something you don't know if you keep on doing what you do know" (Maisel, 1974 p. 5).

searching   On release of the stagnation which has occurred in the organism, the search begins for more effective alternatives through exploration in dance movement and the development of what holds promise. In all therapies much depends on the clients' courage to shed the old and harness the new and unfamiliar. In dance even greater risks have to be taken because of its demands on mind *and* body.

resistance   Resistance must be expected. Gelb says: "Fear is the biggest block to learning in an integral way" (p. 98). Many people cling to their symptoms because they fear that letting them go would commit them to facing what they are afraid to cope with.

We do take into account however that certain habits, though they have become damaging physically or psychically, may have been adopted initially as a protective measure. They still might be useful in certain circumstances; in that case it is a matter of learning to control the habit rather than be controlled by it.

body awareness "The body is our instrument for fulfilling our purpose on earth. This instrument can be coarse and dull or finely tuned and receptive—the choice is ours" (Gelb, p. 35). What matters is not whether we are skinny or round, tall or short, but gaining a realistic recognition of where we are in our bodies, how we need to care for them and what they can do for us.

physical conditions

This is vitally important for those with primarily physical conditions, who are often bound by an unrealistic perception of their bodies, which forms a block to change. For them the way into learning is to take a new look at themselves and their whole situation. Such involvement, where possible, will pave the way for improvement which may well exceed all previous expectations (see Appendix 3, Body Image).

psychical disturbances

The course that learning will take in cases of primarily psychical disturbances is somewhat different. In the first instance, the client has to learn to *put the mind into the body*. In that way he will *own* the issue physically. He will experience grief, anger, fear, in his bones, muscles and skin. Learning to put the mind into the body often takes time, yet is in itself therapeutic. Many clients entering therapy suffer from dissociation of body and mind. Allowing thoughts and feelings to flow through the body so that they are experienced in shape and motion can be exceedingly difficult. Yet it is a necessary way towards understanding one's inner state. On the other hand, clients with dance experience may have acquired the habit of "acting out" rather than feeling out bodily, what plagues them. For such clients the path to learning often proves to be more difficult than for the novice because they have to shed their tendency towards dramatizing first.

In our method we draw on the wisdom of the body: we trust the body's own mode of knowing, we encourage it to "speak its mind."

choice

Change, when it occurs, must take place by choice. Clients will be acquainted with movements other than their habitual ones, to experiment with and to test; in the case of a physical problem, perhaps alternative ways of using crutches, or if the desired change is psychical, trying out different movement qualities. Options provide the basis for making responsible choices.[4] As we have pointed out, the client may need to temporarily retain a habitual movement pattern, unsound as it might be. We would not expect him to let go of it before he has discovered that there are other and better ways to operate. The habitual way may, as previously stated, be useful in certain situations but should not dominate his actions in all circumstances. For example, one should be able to choose whether to respond directly or indirectly to an aggressive approach. If the habitual response has been to withdraw and one does so in spite of the fact that one would like to confront the aggressor, then resentment, frustration and anger build up and can lead to psychophysical disturbances. Being able to choose is the key issue.

practice

Body learning, like any other form of learning, makes little or no progress without practice. Practice should become a condition of the dance therapy contract. If for some reason the clients are themselves unable to take on the responsibility for practising, assistance from carers would be sought. Home practices* themselves are always body oriented. Their main objectives are to establish *continuity* and to *reinforce* the therapeutic work. Practising gives clients confidence in themselves and in the therapy. There is no better way to increase motivation.

evidence of change

Experience has taught us not to trust that progress has been made unless visible changes in bodyshape and motion are occurring, no matter how convincing the clients' verbal assurances may sound. Watzlawick, Weakland and Fisch (1974) devoted an entire work to the issue of change. The main focus of their enquiry was directed towards discovering why an intolerable situation in which an individual or a group is caught continues in spite of strenuous attempts to break free. The authors posed two dominant questions: "How does this undesirable situation persist?" and "What is required to change it?" (p. 2). Their research led them into the field of mathematics and from their findings they drew conclusions applicable to the human situation. They postulated that "there

---

*See Method on p. 58 and p. 59.

are two different types of change: one that occurs *within a given system* [italics added] which in itself remains unchanged, and one whose occurrence *changes the system itself* [italics added]" (p. 10). They refer to the former, the change within the system, as "*first order change* [italics added]" and "the change to an altogether different state . . . as *second order change* [italics added]" (p. 10), concluding that only a change in the system itself would be decisive.

In the context of our work, the system we deal with is the human organism. We, too, differentiate between first and second order change. Change of the second order, in terms of dance therapy, is change that becomes evident *physically.* Before we trust the changes are under way, let alone that they have occurred, we must see them "in the flesh." This goes without saying where physical problems are concerned but, to the best of our knowledge, has so far not been a criterion for change in psychotherapeutic work. Yet we are certain that while the body retains its laxity, tension, stoop or twist, the mind is bound to slip back into its accustomed frame which holds the problems in place. There has only been a first order change.

transformation Changes often announce themselves by infinitesimal shifts in body attitude which, if recognised and reinforced, may in time lead to deeper transformations. The term "transformation" is generally used to describe an inner change, yet we have also observed this phenomenon in instances of physical problems. At a certain moment a client finds the "right" alignment, the "right" way to use crutches, the "right" way of attaining balance. A change of the second order has occurred and *a new and more effective configuration has been found.*

maintaining the change Fish (in Pentony 1981) sees the therapeutic process consisting of the Exploratory Phase, the Healing Ritual and Maintaining the Cure (p. 57). We prefer to call the third phase *Maintaining the Change.* This aspect of the therapeutic process has rarely been discussed, yet we regard it as an indispensable continuation of the therapy itself. Maintaining the change requires application in everyday life of what has been learned until it is fully integrated. Changes need fostering. We like to remind ourselves of the saying "Old habits die hard." And we add: *They readily resurrect!* This is why maintenance of the change is essential.

V. GIVING FORM TO EXPRESSIVE MATERIAL

The burgeoning of *expressive* dance which gave rise to the eventual function of dance as therapy in modern society, was due to those artists who liberated dance from its artificiality at the turn of the century.

Isadora Duncan

At the headwaters of this flow of change was undoubtedly Isadora Duncan. She fought a passionate and often painful battle for freedom of expression in dance. Her personal eccentricies at times overshadowed the credit she deserves for her revolutionary ideas not only for dance, but for education, ethics, and the rights of women. Many of her disciples, attracted merely by her flowing Greek tunics and her "love of the beautiful," did not understand her true worth. They misinterpreted her rejection of the inflexible rules established by the classical ballet as being a rejection of any kind of control.

In fact, Isadora Duncan was by no means in favour of a *laissez-faire* approach to dance. While she brought back its spontaneity she did not neglect its form. The difference was that she arrived at it organically in the process of creation. She could rely on her great gift to achieve a balance between freedom and discipline. She spent hours working in front of her mirror, seeking to discover which configuration of body line and shape looked and felt right for what she wanted to express. But Duncan remained an isolated phenomenon despite the fact that her sister Elizabeth carried on teaching her method.

The times though were ripe for change. Independently from Duncan came a stream of individual dance artists. The most prominent in Europe were Mary Wigman,

Gertrud Bodenwieser, Kurt Joos and Harald Kreutzberg; and in America, Ted Shawn, Martha Graham, Doris Humphrey and José Limon. They broke with tradition and danced about issues that mattered politically, socially and psychologically, in a style that reflected their particular personalities.

While "The New Dance," as Bodenwieser referred to it,[5] progressed along its course, *improvisation* became an integral element. Its practice was added to dance training (and also to music teaching through the influence of Emile Jaques-Dalcroze[6]). Furthermore, it became established as the creative tool of the choreographic process.

Expressionism in dance   And so as dance aligned itself with the expressionist movement in the other arts, it regained its humanity. The expression of emotion and feelings became its driving force.

Suzanne Langer on the language of art   Suzanne Langer in "The Cultural Importance of the Arts" in *Aesthetics and the Problem of Education* (1971) gives a convincing reason for the natural flow from inner experience to expressive movement. She writes: "There is . . . an important part of reality that is quite inaccessible to the formative influence of language: That is the realm of so called inner experience, the life of feeling and emotion" (p. 90). The discursive nature of language, therefore, does not do justice to the "natural form of feeling." Feelings create their own type of patterns which are different from, but no less discernible than, those of language. As Langer says: "It is I think, this dynamic pattern [of feelings] that finds its formal expression in the arts" (p. 91).

It seems to us that the terms emotion and feeling are often used interchangeably. We feel it is important to distinguish between them. In our search for a differentiation we discovered an illuminating definition by the contemporary writer and poet Vincent Buckley in his book *Poetry and Morality* (1959):

Vincent Buckley on emotion and feeling

"The difference between *emotion* and *feeling* would seem to be that the former is simply a temporary response to experience, while the latter is something by which the person becomes attached to actuality. It is thus both a WAY of experiencing the actual world, and a capacity for keeping that experience constant" (p. 114).

To expand on this in our own words: emotions have the tendency to fluctuate, or to well up and subside completely. Emotions can transform into feelings if they reach a kind of plateau and become integrated with a person's way of being. From the stability of this plateau, one can contemplate emotions, accept them as part of experience and yet not be swept away.

the choreographic process

Early this century dancers such as Martha Graham were well aware that dance in its truest form could become "a revelation of the inner landscape which is man's heart"[7] and that achieving this insight demanded deep commitment, invariably involving its creators in a long inner struggle with their material. In working through the conflicts and meeting the demands made by the creative process itself, dancers experienced a growing sense of release from which they emerged "cleansed," refreshed and edified.

dance as catharsis

Recognition of two of dance's most powerful elements, its expressive quality and its potential to become cathartic, awakened in a number of dance artists the realization that dance could be of considerable benefit to patients suffering from psychic disturbances. In the USA Marian Chace,[8] Trudi Schoop, Jerri Salkin, Liljan Espenak were among those in the forefront. Some psychiatrists responded positively to their proposals and offered invitations to conduct programs in various mental health institutions.

It is interesting to note that in the transfer of dance into the psychiatric domain two further elements which make dance what it is, were often left behind: The *body* and *form.* Maybe the early therapists, being dancers themselves, took the body for granted as it had been trained to serve

them well. It seems that it was the psyche and its disturbances which captured their imagination. What surprises
though is that no emphasis was placed on the *forming of
expressive material,* though all dancers who create their
own choreography (as all the pioneers did) know that in
order to come to grips with an idea it needs to be *worked
through.* When dance entered the psychotherapeutic
domain, the working-through, the crux of the process,
was mainly conducted verbally with some variations.
This model is still in use today.

*reflection and
resolution
through dance*

In our approach a different course of action is taken.
We believe that the material which arises in the improvisation must be worked through, that is be shaped and
re–shaped in dance. In struggling to give it form one
disentangles and illuminates what has been experienced.
Not to do so in action deprives clients of the full value of
the dance.

To change horses in midstream, to move from engagement in a nonverbal creative mode to a verbal discourse
is not giving dance its due, and what is equally important,
it interrupts the flow. Words will present themselves
when the time is ripe, which is not before new under-
standings have been given form in the act of dancing. To
leave off when movements are fuzzy and incomplete will
neither bring about understanding nor change. *Clarity* is
vital.[9]

*choreographic
aspect*

While working with clients on giving form to expressive
material, similarities with the choreographic process are
undeniable.* At the same time the pronounced differences have to be understood: a client works for *himself,* not
for an audience. He does not proclaim a message; he need
not be concerned with matters of performing and project-
ing. He selects and clarifies *to understand himself and his
condition.* Flashes of awareness reward him for his labor.

ritual

Clarity and a sense of purpose in movement can be
helped along by imagining it to be part of a ritual.

*See Appendix 2.

Rituals require that we strip the action down to its essentials. The precision a ritual demands will bring the client closer to the core of the problem.

A description of the practical application of giving form to expressive material is provided in the DEDUCTIVE APPROACH which we consider to be primarily suited to clients with psychical problems. In a less extensive way it can serve as an addition to the INDUCTIVE APPROACH if and when the guided physical phases flow on to dance exploration (see Chapter 4).

NOTES

1. We make a clear distinction between the *general therapeutic effect* which may be gained from becoming sensitively, mindfully and imaginatively involved in any form of dance, be it folk, ballroom, ballet, modern or improvisational, and *therapy as rehabilitation* and *where possible restoration* of physical and psychical health. All creative activity which absorbs us and feels rewarding could be classed as therapeutic in the sense of taking us out of the humdrum of everyday existence and making us feel better, richer and more "together." We suggest however that the appropriate term for this kind of pursuit is *recreation* for which Yukic (1970) has contributed an enlightened definition:

    "Recreation is an act or experience, selected by the individual during his leisuretime, to meet a personal want or desire, primarily for his own satisfaction" (p. 5).

    In comparison, therapy as we understand it, refers to work with clients who cannot deal with specific physical and/or psychical conditions without professional assistance.

2. Liljan Espenak (1905–1988) was a pioneer in the field of dance therapy. She wrote *Dance Therapy, Theory and Application* (published 1981) as well as numerous papers on the subject. In addition to being a practising dance therapist she was the first teacher of dance therapy at college level (New York Medical College 1968) and lectured world wide. She rejected the terms *patient* or *client* for the people she worked with, preferring to call them *students*.

3. F. Mathias Alexander (1869–1955) developed a system of psycho-physical re-education known today as the Alexander Technique. He published four books: *Man's Supreme Inheritance, Constructive Conscious Control of the Individual, The Use of the Self* and *The Universal Constant in Living.*

4. Mary Whitehouse, pioneer Jungian dance therapist, had this to say about change: "Change can happen and development can take place through the discovery of unused and previously unavailable qualities of movement. For

instance, something as simple but as basic as large, strong, assertive action in a forward direction can be built up gradually from a walk, and coaxed, not commanded, from the timid, self-apologetic ones. The experience of this new quality of movement provides a change in feeling, another dimension of the Self. Change can also take place through the discovery of previously unavailable feelings" (Whitehouse, 1969, p. 274).

5. It became the title of her book *The New Dance* published posthumously by Marie and Eric Cuckson, 1970.

6. Emile Jaques-Dalcroze, Swiss music educator (1865–1950).

7. Spoken by Graham in the commentary to the film of her choreographic work "Diversion of Angels" from the series: *Dance in America*, Martha Graham Company, Part 2, Bloomington Indiana Audio Visual Center, published by WNET 1976.

8. Marian Chace stood out as a dance therapist who paid careful attention to the role of the body. She recognised that psychical disturbances always had a physical counterpart, a recognition she took full account of in her therapeutic work. She rated inner awareness, the sensing of movement itself, as an indispensable facet of therapeutic dance.

    As with most of the dance therapists of her era, Chace's dominant goal was for clients to learn to express themselves through dance movement and by doing so bring issues to be dealt with to the surface.

    It appears that since that time the important role of the body in dance therapy has faded into the background.

9. Clarity and precision are dependent on factors such as paying attention to a movement's point of departure, its pathway and its destination (SPACE) and being clear about its dynamic quality (TIME and ENERGY FLOW). It also requires concern with punctuation and phrasing.

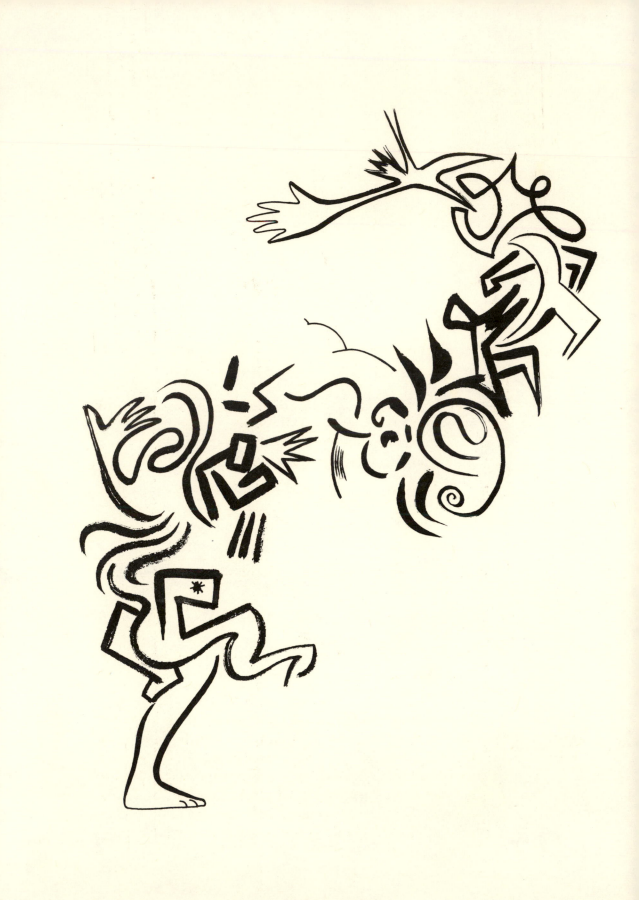

Chapter 4

THE DANCE THERAPEUTIC PROCESS

"Putting dance back into the body as a moment by moment sensation is part of the voyage, is part of the revolution."
Erick Hawkins in *The Body Is A Clear Place,* 1992, p. 22.

I. OBSERVATION AND APPRAISAL

People always present themselves in SHAPE and MOTION. They really have no other way. To us as therapists shape and motion represent the clients' psychophysical state. This provides the basis for our therapeutic work which is always through the body.

"There's language in her eye, her cheek, her lip,
Nay, her foot speaks; her wanton spirits look out
At every joint and motive of her body."

William Shakespeare, *Troilus and Cressida* IV, v. 55

It follows then that in our method *observation and appraisal* are essential in order to:

(a) understand and assess the person's psychophysical condition,
(b) work out a programme of both short- and long-term goals, and
(c) monitor progress.

initial observations
In the first instance we observe the way clients meet us; noting their degree of hesitancy, confidence or self consciousness, how they hold their bodies (posture), how they walk (locomotion), what gestures they use. We look at facial expression. We pay attention to the way they talk and whether they are voluble or reticent. We note whether they seem comfortable or out of touch with their bodies.

37

There is also information to be gleaned from the clients' own reporting. The more clues we pick up, the better will be the picture we form of the person at that particular time:

For the dance therapist gestures are as important a communication as words are for the verbal therapist.

What movement communicates is sensitively expressed by Mary Whitehouse (1969):

> "Our movement is our *behaviour;* there is a direct connection between what we are like and how we move. Distortion, tension, and deadness in our movement is distortion, tension, and deadness in ourselves" (p. 274).

movement behaviour

Eric Berne (1976) is adamant about the necessity to observe the client's movement behaviours down to the smallest detail for these are indicative of the patient's "script." Only if the patient gets " 'out of his script' can he emerge as a person capable of autonomous vitality, fulfillment and citizenship." Berne also states categorically that "whatever theoretical approach he is using (the therapist) is to observe every movement of every muscle, of every patient during every second . . . " (p. 278).

Similarly, Rollo May (1969): "When a patient comes in the door of my consulting room intentionality* is is expressed in his way of walking, his gestures; does he lean toward me or away? Does he talk with a *half closed mouth.* " May goes on to say, "Not only in the therapeutic hour but in real life as well, our communication has, much more than we are aware of it, *the subtle character of the dance* [italics added], the meaning communicated by virtue of the forms we continuously create by our bodily movements" (p. 241).

From such first impressions we proceed to a more systematic appraisal.

specific observations

First, we need to find out where in the body the disturbance is located: is it confined to one place or spread over wider areas? We draw information from the articu-

*See Chapter 1, note 8.

lation of body parts, the coordination of body movements, and how the person moves in terms of SPACE, TIME and ENERGY FLOW (see pp. 40, 41). We also note which body parts clients favour and we make a distinction between clients' everyday body language and their choice of movement qualities when they are dancing.

body activities   Observation of body activities[1] in dance provides information on the client's abilities or limitations to involve his body in action. Arm and hand gestures are dominant in most cases, not surprisingly since we move them in a variety of ways in day-to-day living. The torso and neck tend to remain rigid, so do shoulders. Legs and feet are mostly restricted to locomotion and weight support. Fingers and toes rarely take part in undirected movement experiments. Hip movements range from pronounced swaying to total rigidity. When dancing, clients need much encouragement to use elevation, turning, falling. Some of these activities may, of course, be totally outside certain clients' scope. Yet one needs to be quite sure whether the clients are really physically unable to do the movements or whether anxiety or resistance prevents them from making the attempt.

We observe the degree of ease with which clients who are new to dance respond to the movement experiments being offered. For instance, one client may enjoy doing quick and strong movements rather than sustained slow ones. Another may like moving about freely in space but may be uncomfortable staying in one place.

We note all these characteristics in order to gain a picture of the person's movement preferences.

attitudinal characteristics   Throughout the course of the therapy we also consider attitudinal characteristics such as:

- discrepancies between physical and verbal messages
- motivation
- a sense of purpose when engaged in movement
- taking responsibility for one's own condition
- balance of spontaneity and control

- quality of physical presence
- attentiveness
- inner participation
- risk taking

quality of movement

In our observation of the quality of motion, we draw on the fundamental principles identified by RUDOLF LABAN* without applying Laban Movement Analysis in a formal manner. Laban successfully *grounded* dance by planting it firmly in the field of movement itself, establishing it as a discipline in its own right.

Laban refers to dance as the *language of action,* and postulates that every movement, such as an extension or contraction, is an experience in itself and does not need to have expressive connotations.

As other movement and dance specialists have done, we allow ourselves to interpret Laban's work with quite some degree of freedom. Yet we do not contradict any of his basic teachings, as we believe there is no better foundation than Laban's for defining movement, wherever it occurs.

Use of Laban terminology

We use Laban's qualification of progress in SPACE as being either *direct* or *indirect.* We retain *sudden* and *sustained* as contrasting characteristics of a movement's release in TIME. Our interpretation of Laban's concept of WEIGHT differs in the sense that we do not consider WEIGHT to be the determining factor in producing motion. Laban himself states (1960) "that the *weight* of the body, or any of its parts, can be lifted and carried into a certain direction of *space* and this process takes a certain amount of *time...* " (pp. 22–23). This implies that weight in itself is not a motion factor. In our understanding, movement is created by the amount of ENERGY that is being released, and we characterise it as being either *high* or *low.* While Laban does not list energy as one of the four motion factors (SPACE, TIME,

*See Note 8 in Preface.

WEIGHT & FLOW), he certainly refers to energy as the principle that generates movement.

"The driving force of the movement is the *energy* developed by a process of combustion within the organs of the body. The fuel consumed in the process is food. There is no doubt about the purely physical character of the production of energy and its transformation into movement" (p. 22).

We accept Laban's description of FLOW as being *bound* or *free*. However, we see FLOW as being inseparable from ENERGY. We have drawn these two principles together because we consider the flow of energy forms the stuff of movement itself, ENERGY FLOW *is* motion.[2]

As well as placing importance on the polarities in each of the movement elements, we take great care not to overlook the significance of gradations in between. In addition, the movers' responses to the elements are of importance. These responses are characterised by either giving oneself over to the experiences of SPACE, TIME and ENERGY FLOW, that is letting them act on one: this Laban calls "indulging;" controlling, and taking charge of them, Laban calls "fighting" (pp. 23–24, 59–75). An example of "indulging" could be to imagine no limits to space with time and energy uncontrolled; in contrast, "fighting" would create a precise pattern in time and space and control the flow of energy.

Laban's effort actions   In summary then, we observe a movement's FLOW of ENERGY in SPACE and TIME. We draw on Laban's eight EFFORT ACTIONS (punch, slash, press, wring, dab, flick, glide, float) as reference points to describe a client's movement behaviour. However, we replace Laban's element of WEIGHT with ours of ENERGY FLOW.[3] In doing so we do not contradict Laban who said, "certain elementary actions have a natural tendency towards 'free flow,' for example, *slashing* in which the flow of movement is suddenly and energetically released; others, for example, *pressing* require restraint of flow so that the movement can be stopped at any given moment" (1960,

p. 21). In broad terms we might characterise a person as a "floater" or "puncher," but at the same time we take note of the subtle variations inherent in each one of the effort actions.

shape

In the context of appraisal we see that *body shape* in stillness holds within it all the ingredients of *the motion which preceded it.** For example, a sharp-edged shape is the result of sudden/direct high-energy motion, while a sustained/indirect low-energy movement will lead to soft and rounded outlines.

People move from shape to shape as they conduct their daily lives. Some never pause. Their shapes are fluid and indistinct. Others hardly change the shape of the body in motion. We usually describe them as "stiff." (In extreme cases, as in cataleptic states, shape takes over.) Body shapes, their size, contour, differentiation and texture, in stillness and in motion, represent the person in a variety of aspects. This calls for acute attention.

posture

Adult posture is the outcome of genetic and environmental factors, combined with attitudes an individual adopts in the course of growing up. (Posture may also be the result of irreversible damage to the organism.)

At all stages of our life, posture is a determining factor in our movement behaviour and vice versa. (1) For instance, a person who is trapped in a bowed twisted posture is the product of habitual tense twisted movement with a downward orientation. (2) There is an optimal way for the body to be aligned so that, with a minimum of stress, it can respond to the demands which life places on the organism. Such organisation of muscles, ligaments and joints, would give access to the widest possible range of mobility as well as strength. In actual fact, however, there are often limitations on the way the organism develops. People who come into therapy have reached a stage where the effective functioning of the organism is no longer possible.

---

*This can readily be observed by pressing the pause button while watching videotaped motion.

shadow movements	Laban maintained that in movement behaviour people give two types of signals: those that are intentional, to underline the spoken word, for instance, and those which are unintentional, in response to unconscious experiences. The latter he refers to as "shadow movements" which he considers highly significant when interpreting a person's manner of moving.
movement modes	In ordinary behaviour as well as in dance, we recognise that people have individual *modes of moving,* modes which have developed in the process of growing up and are composed, like everything else in human development, of a mixture of nature and nurture.[4]
major and minor modes	A well-balanced person will have a *major* mode of moving which feels comfortable and suits her, as well as many *minor* modes adopted on different occasions and in order to perform different tasks. To be effective, our habitual or major way of moving needs to remain flexible.
modulations	We pay attention to the way people *modulate* their movements to suit the action they are engaged in, using energy either in short spurts or in a sustained manner. We note whether a person relaxes when pausing or holds on tight. The latter points to overcontrol of energy flow. Lack of control leads to disorganised behaviour and in extreme cases to breakdown. The desired goal is of course to use control appropriately. Laban describes this as a "rational control of strength resources" (1960 p. 12).
kinetic identification	All observation is accomplished by means of *kinetic empathy.* Naturally we perceive motion through our eyes, but unless we let this perception flow on into the body so that we experience it kinetically, we cannot identify with it. And because of the inseparability of body and mind, *kinetic identification* is mandatory for the psychophysical understanding of the clients' condition.
self observation	Once our clients have become familiar with the language of dance, we may introduce the idea of *self observation* for identifying areas of the body which house emotional conflicts, or indicate physical disturbances. As self obser-

vation may be threatening, the client needs to be ready to take that step. When looking at themselves, (in the mirror or on videotape), clients learn to take stock of 'what their bodies can tell them,' realising that the body reflects a person's assets as well as problem areas. Once clients feel safe, self assessment gives them a useful opportunity to become constructively involved in the choice of further therapeutic action.

II. METHOD

INTRODUCTION

Our model of dance therapy incorporates two complementary approaches:

INDUCTIVE and DEDUCTIVE[5]

differences between INDUCTIVE and DEDUCTIVE approach

In the INDUCTIVE approach we work from the individual movement to the whole dance. In the DEDUCTIVE we begin with the whole dance and subsequently explore its parts.

The INDUCTIVE approach allows for a gradual entry into dance and will be suitable for those whose problems are largely physical, although it may be the preferred option for any other type of client.

The DEDUCTIVE approach is suitable for those clients with psychical problems who have a background in dance, drama or music, or who possess an innate ability to express themselves in movement.

The two approaches are not mutually exclusive, however. They may alternate from session to session, or even within one session, depending on what emerges during the therapy.

One could perhaps describe the therapeutic process as a continuum between INDUCTION and DEDUCTION in the shape of two intertwining spirals. Where the therapy starts, in which direction it proceeds or crosses over from one to the other, will depend on the need of the moment.

The examples of strategies we give in the following sections have either been found useful with clients and/or explored with colleagues in dance therapy workshops. At times they have been deduced from such educational, recreational or pure dance pursuits which unmistakably indicated connections with dance therapy.

(a) INDUCTIVE APPROACH

working with physical problems

With clients who present mainly physical problems we develop practices which address themselves to the specific needs of the body.[6] Before this can be done, an overall tuning-up of the body is necessary. Sometimes a "warm-up" is required, sometimes a "cool-down." The action might be to stimulate, "defrost" or soothe.

preliminary practices

No matter what preliminary actions are being taken a *sensitising* of the body is mandatory.

Sensitising is a strategy for body awareness, for full body participation and for developing a realistic body image.* We make appropriate movement suggestions to accomplish any of these introductory moves such as brushing, tapping, shaking, circling, airing and "breathing" with different body parts and body areas.

Or, we may encourage clients to discover and develop their own actions. At the same time we will insist that all practices are performed with sensitivity, mindfulness and imagination, i.e. *in the dance mode.* To initiate greater body-mind involvement, we make suggestions such as "Take your mind into your body, feel out your body from top to toe."

In the course of preliminary practices, areas of the body which are somewhat out of harmony with the rest, will be discovered.

disharmonies

These disharmonies may manifest themselves as resisting movement, or on the other hand, a body part may appear out of control.[7] Body areas may seem overworked, overprotected, vulnerable, painful or weak.

---

*See Appendix 3.

overall adjustment   While attending to an affected body part, we also take into account its relationship to the whole body and devise practices for overall adjustment.[8] Provided we remain in the orbit of dance, body-oriented practices will invariably bring about associations with feeling states which can be subsequently explored.

development   If, for example, a client demonstrates rigidity located in the thoracic region of the spine, we will begin with an exercise to mobilise this specific area and, if appropriate, explore a number of variations. With one or two of these exercises as a starting point we now proceed to develop a movement sequence in which the upper back mobilisation is followed by a pelvic articulation (which takes in the lumbar region) and concludes with an extension and circling of the neck. Sequences of this nature are valuable because they address themselves to the interaction between related areas of the body and add interest and enjoyment to the practices themselves.

compensatory practices   If part or all of one side of the body is causing the disturbance and consequently becomes central to the remedial work, we would find it necessary to add some compensatory movements for the corresponding area on the other side of the body. We work on the principle that any local disturbance results in a structural imbalance, and we offer practices to reintegrate the troublesome part into the system as far as feasible.

Variations of rhythm, space patterns and the degree of energy flow broaden and deepen the therapeutic effect.

use of music   Music, carefully chosen, can make the dance experience doubly pleasurable. Once suitable music has been found we encourage clients to use it for practising. If they are enterprising they can create their own variations on a given sequence, provided they keep its major objective in mind. This could perhaps, in the case of the example given above, lead the client to an improvisation "around the lumbar region" for which a new piece of music would probably be more appropriate.

But here comes a caution! In attempting to match the rhythm and keep up with the speed of the music, one easily slips into inaccuracies in the execution of the practice, that invariably do more harm than good. (See more about use of music this chapter, pp. 61–63.)

working with psychosomatic conditions When dealing with psychosomatic conditions, we initially address the somatic symptom in the manner just described for a primarily physical problem. Psychical material, which surfaces during the course of the physical work, points to the origins of the clients' symptoms and gradually leads to recognition of the multifaceted nature of their condition.

understanding psychosomatic connections As the therapy progresses and the client's obsessive concern with what he considers to be his purely physical problem fades, he will start to talk about the links he discovers between his physical condition and its psychical origin. This understanding of the reality of the psychophysical connection is the turning point at which the therapy enters a deeper, more holistic stage. Feelings expressed in words are now taken back into the body and experienced dynamically in movement. Fear, for example, may be paralysing, or it may make you run. In the experience of joy, one may choose stillness or whirling or leaping. Feelings also take on shapes. Anger may be sensed as being bulky or thin, and in action be expressed in thumps or stabs. Confusion is likely to distort the body and fragment its movements. Clients' responses vary and are unpredictable.

pure movements giving rise to emotions The INDUCTIVE approach allows clients to let feelings flow into movement when they are ready. Since movements in themselves need have no emotional connotations and clients are not pushed "to express themselves" they enter movement exploration without undue tension or nervousness.

In the progression from movement for movement's sake to expressive movement, the opening of the arms may trigger off a sense of relief, or it may become a plea for help. Closing the arms may be comforting or defensive. Advancing may initiate feelings either of welcoming or attacking. Retreating may evoke disappointment or fear. It is well known that movement is not only a response to feeling but also creates feeling states. In the training of soldiers, specific movements are used to heighten feelings of aggression. The mother gently rocking her child is calming the baby and herself. We make use of such movement effects in our therapy.

However, our suggestions or questions as to what one or the other movement may mean to the client are likely to be ignored early on but will gradually elicit responses. These responses, of course, vary considerably from person to person and within persons themselves at different times. Transitions into expressiveness often require considerable guidance, as the discovery of hitherto suppressed emotions can become an overpowering experience.

In the course of a session we create movement sequences with the client by giving him suggestions for developing expressive improvisations, provided, of course, that the client is not intimidated by the thought of such experiments. While doing so we ensure that the aesthetic component is not disregarded or overshadowed by the physical and emotional aspects.

In working with sequences we have found it useful to ask ourselves a number of questions such as:

> What were the aims of the sequence?
> Have the aims been achieved?
> Did the sequence meet the objectives in terms of:
> * overall awareness of and attention to the body?
> * focussing on the area under consideration?
> * the physical and psychical needs of the clients?

Sequences which have evolved in the course of a session often become the basis for practising at home.* (See CONCEPTUAL FRAMEWORK, p. 27.)

---

*Only when the client fully understands all aspects of a practice may it be chosen to be his home practice.

When it comes to the end of a session, which is when talk about home practice usually takes place, we will ensure that the client reaches a state of comparative comfort and leaves confident that further growth is possible.

clients identifying own objective

Another inductive path which could be taken begins with a statement by clients about the kind of changes they want to bring about and what they want to achieve. For example: a client who considers himself clumsy or may have even been criticised by his boss for it, wishes to improve his coordination; another expresses the opinion that his failures are due to an erratic way of approaching people, and seeks to improve his communication skills; yet another wants to adopt a less agitated, more controlled and decisive attitude.

movement experiments

In response to the clients' stated needs and our observation of their everyday movement behaviour, we acquaint them, through experimentation, with movement qualities different from their habitual ones. We link these movement experiments to exercises which will release their habitual body posture and allow for a greater freedom of motion.

working with a physical problem

For example, we worked with a client who suffered from chronic neck and shoulder pain which was obvious from the tension displayed in that part of her body. The question which arose was the possible relationship between the body attitude and the pain: was the pain the cause of the posture, the posture the cause of the pain or how much did each contribute to the problem?

The work began by experimenting with gentle movements to release the observed tension. These included swaying, undulating, rippling, rising, sinking and rotating of the affected area. We then selected the movements which were felt to be the most appropriate and built a sequence around them. Development continued quite organically by letting the movement flow down to the rib cage and eventually to the base of the spine. A dance improvisation grew out of the functional and qualitative nature of the practice. The recognition that the problem may in fact have originated in the lower back gave us a starting point for the next session. We also became aware that most likely a psychical component contributed to the painful condition.

No matter what symptom clients present, we draw their attention to the fact that merely *adopting* a different posture or quality of motion is not enough. Any true changes have to come from within and reach every part of the body. The whole organism must participate to support the desired transformation, and this can only be achieved by means of practice.

choosing alternative movement modes

Before the choice of a new movement mode is made the client will have experienced numerous alternatives, and will be well on the way to discarding the habitual obstructive posture. The client's final decision is made on the basis of what feels right for him. The client modifies behaviour by choice! Improvising in the manner of the newly acquired movement mode supports the desired change. Specific home practices consolidate the learning that has taken place in sessions.

examples of working with psychical disturbances

In some clients with psychical disturbances, the connection between body and mind is readily observable by the type of movements that accompany a spoken report. Take, for example, a desperate gripping of the head while the body is in the act of bending down. These shape and movement signals provide *physical* starting points for *inductive* therapy. Our response to these signals depends to some extent on intuition as well as on our assessment of the complaint. In the above instance we would place our hands on those of the client, slightly reinforcing the grip on the head and increasing the forward bend during an exhalation of breath, then reducing the pressure on the head to gently open the curved body-shape during inhalation. As breathing continues, the distance travelled in the opening out increases. The hands may gradually detach from the head during inhalation, while during exhalation the degree of tension and the length of the return journey decreases. The sequence may conclude with a deeper breath, a sigh of release, then a pause in the open shape.

If we feel that the client wishes to retain his initial bowed shape, rocking, rising and sinking while breathing with the client in synchrony might be more welcome. A client who is not expressing his emotional state in his body shape (as described in our previous example), can, with assistance, be induced to do so. Appropriate questions will elicit verbal responses as to how the client is feeling, which, however, we redirect back to the body and we now help him to express these feelings in body shapes. In the process of this strategy a number of shapes are discovered, thereby forming a sequence, and without noticing it the client has started to dance!

the role of words

Verbal accompaniment seems to be indispensable in the early stages of inductive work. Words are one way of maximising the potential of dance experience, drawing increased attention to what the movement has to offer. The combination of words with movement may lead clients to discover more easily the rudiments of a thera-peutic dance. (See Use of Language, this chapter, pp. 59–61.)

It would be inappropriate to make predictions as to how any such dance would develop, since this depends on so many variables: the stage of the therapy, the rapport between client and therapist, and the client's responses. To help clients use movement more fully, coherently and courageously, *we extend their movement vocabulary and range of movement qualities.* In saying that, it becomes obvious that we believe a considerable aspect of dance therapy (or any therapy) requires *teaching*.

teaching strategies

As part of teaching we may introduce dance practices by means of mirroring.

In **mirroring** two people face one another, taking turns to copy the other's actions. This is an inductive strategy which has been popular in both drama and dance teaching. In our work we consider mirroring is not only an effective way of assisting a client to become acquainted with another's dance movements, but also of developing an awareness of his own individual way of moving. (See *GROUP WORK* this chapter, pp. 65–67.) We also make sure that clients *internalise* the mirrored movements, centering them in their own bodies. We have found that unless this happens mirroring contributes little if anything to the therapy.

If the client has mirrored the therapist, who has of course chosen movements advisedly, the therapist may ask:

> "Which movements made you feel different?"
> "Which felt most comforting?"
> "Which movements would you like to do again?"

As soon as possible the client is encouraged to take the lead, which the therapist follows. This reinforces clients' often timid attempts and also helps them make their movement patterns clearer. As they gain confidence, the act of mirroring may develop into a duet, with both taking an equal role. The therapist, however, remains attentive to opportunities for widening the parameters of the experience.

Sculpting, a more body-oriented strategy, is also very useful for clients with physical problems. Here, the therapist places himself behind the client, both facing the same direction. Exerting gentle pressure on the client's body while moving, the therapist simultaneously leads and supports. In breaking through the constraints of habitual movement patterns and for relearning lost physical skills (e.g. walking, balancing), *sculpting* is an invaluable way of teaching.

less threatening forms of partnering

In dance therapy, becoming a partner in the actions is far preferable to demonstrating. However, there are clients who feel uncomfortable about close physical proximity, in which case we may make the interaction less threatening by using a scarf or length of cloth as a link. For some, though, their discomfort may prove the catalyst for them to start experimenting on their own. This, from a psychological point of view, is at least as productive as yielding to being shaped or mirrored.

An important therapeutic strategy is the setting of **frames** or parameters which set limits to the extent of the client's dance exploration. Establishing a frame offers scope for the clients to make discoveries about where resistances exist. Frames assist the clients to acquaint themselves with unfamiliar movement experiences and to accept or reject them. For instance, we might say, "Slow motion *only* please, sudden movements are *out of bounds*," "Experiment with movements *close to the ground*" or "Use *body gestures only*, don't move into space yet." Such directions often provide the challenge the client needs to overcome his habitual resistance. We appreciate that some clients will break out of the frame when they are not yet ready to cope with the unfamiliar. Others may take delight in the new experience and by delving into it overcome their fears. When they are ready they may let the frame dissolve as they enter into another movement mode or choose to relax and rest.

A strategy which has proved valuable for clients with psychosomatic or psychical disturbances may be initiated as follows:

owning the feeling state

"Let the issue/discomfort/pain/confusion travel systematically through every part of your body. Let it ebb and flow through every cell. This will help you to fully own it, to make it more real."

Owning the issue is the first step towards being able to work with it.

Here is a proposed development for adventurous clients:

expanding the exploration

"Now let the mood that flows through your body take you into space. Be open to what the body may tell you to do. For example, move along the floor (SPACE), gather speed (TIME), increase the amount of ENERGY FLOW while crawling, running, leaping, kicking, swinging. In the course of this exploration, shifts may occur in your initial state. Your mood may change. Respond to these changes in the way you move, and in your concluding shape."

stress reduction Suggesting such changes in energy level, speed or other modulations in the way of moving, is a strategy we also use when a client experiences an excessive level of stress. Stress-reducing strategies, more often than not, need to be preceded by their opposites, an intensification in dance of troublesome emotions. (See "Exaggeration" in footnote of *THE DEDUCTIVE APPROACH* this chapter, p. 57.) Over-expansion of energy, or, its opposite, allowing oneself to completely "cave-in," creates a physical need for change, for letting go of the extreme. The principle at work here is similar to that used in relaxation practices, where maximum tensing of muscles precedes the relaxation.

(b) THE DEDUCTIVE APPROACH

improvisation as a means of self-expression
Self-expression by means of improvisation is undoubtedly the first step into the orbit of the DEDUCTIVE approach.[9] Yet it must not remain the be-all and end-all of dance therapy. Explosions, for example, make one feel good. They break the surface and bring buried, untapped, or distorted feelings to the surface, uncovering strengths and weaknesses, fears and hopes, loves and hates. Often much positive psychic material, as well as creativity, lies beneath the rubble and needs release so that it can make its contribution to the work that lies ahead. But once released, it is vitally important to attend to what has emerged by means of *dancing*. If attended to by means of discussion and not through dance, then we have moved out of the domain of dance therapy into verbal therapy.

Conceptualising verbally, we suggest, should affirm what has been worked through in dance. Much can be destroyed by premature talking. In our experience it should be discouraged.

joining with the client
When a person presents with a highly dynamic extroverted attitude expressed in, for instance, sharp, fluttery, restless movements, we would join in his dance and attempt to draw him gradually into a calmer state. In contrast, when the client is very much on guard we again adopt his state and work with him to release his rigidity.

Another strategy, which may be combined with joining the client, is to increase the intensity of his dance. This provides a starting point which holds the promise of a natural, spontaneous release.

recognition of importance of new movements

As the client discovers new movements and/or movement patterns when improvising we will draw attention to certain measures which she may take to make a special movement event "sink in," to recognise its importance, and make it easier to recall.

Suggestions for this may be:

- Selection: "Stay with the (significant) movement. Repeat it."
- Repetition: "Don't throw good movements away. Listen to what they are saying to you!"
- Development: "Would they mean more if you made them bigger, smaller (SHAPE), stronger, softer (ENERGY FLOW), faster, slower (TIME) . . . ?"
- Organisation: "Do the movements link up in some way?"

validation

We help clients to recognise which movements are extraneous and to focus on those that are relevant. Each discovery needs to be tested for its validity, for what it may contribute to the resolution of the problem. These can then be either discarded or taken along, developed and formed.

movement feedback

H'Doubler (1966) discusses the "feedback" which a dancer receives from movement. She says: "The dancer's movements communicate back to him and he must be constantly aware of them and their effect on him" (p. xxv). Garbled feedback will neither be of value in choreography nor in therapy.

clarification

So then, therapist and client will pool their resources to extract essentials, let go of the superfluous, reinforce the positive, investigate emerging leads, until, step by step, clarity comes through, offering the client insights and understanding. This may lead to another dance, reflecting further shifts in attitude. Dance statements of this nature *emerge like pictures* painted at different stages of therapy. From these pictures the client, in collaboration with the therapist, draws information about where he is at that point, and what options there are for change.

review   Discussion with the therapist may follow, yet should not be forced. The client may wish to take the "feel" of the dance away, let it simmer, and request discussion when the time is right.

clarification   If the dance of the client has been rather *undifferentiated*, the working-through process may include, among innumerable others, some of the following comments:

> "It seemed to me that the picture I got from your dance was somewhat blurred. I couldn't quite see whether you searched for something specific or whether you were unsure of what to do and where to go. Could you clarify that?"
> "Does your body remember anything of interest which you might like to go over again, or do you want to wipe it all out and start afresh?"

If, on the other hand, the dance of the client clearly communicated anger, sadness, or confusion, for instance, then we may ask:

> "Would you like to recall any movement or configuration which you felt to be of significance? We could use these to go more deeply into the feeling."

attention to specifics   In our method we receive the dance in its wholeness, but also draw the client's attention to some of its constituents (e.g. prolonged running, a group of erratic movements, periods of stillness). Each constituent represents a different facet of the client's situation. For instance, in the course of one client's improvisation we observed that he had difficulties in using direct pathways in space and in specifically focussing his gaze on a chosen goal. The tactic we chose to help him out of his "meandering" was simply for him to cross the room along straight lines with the eyes directed very purposefully towards a given point. The initial exercise was developed by choosing a number of destinations, pausing before each change of direction to help him concentrate fully on his next move.

Speeding up the action increased the challenge. Alternating curved and angular pathways brought about clarification through contrast. We widened the range of movement possibilities by experimenting with directness using different body parts and body activities. The client was then free to choose how he wanted to conclude the session.

Some may be concerned that such specific instructions may destroy the wholeness of an experience. However, skilfull handling of the situation by the therapist will prevent fragmentation.

If the client has no specific statement to make, the following questions could elicit fruitful responses:

> "Can you describe your dominant movement mode?"
> "Are you satisfied with it? Does it serve you well?"
> "Are you able to modulate it when the need arises?"
> "Which aspects of your mode are useful?"
> "What should be reinforced, what discarded?"
> "Do you consider your movements to be too abrupt, too inhibited, too controlled, too explosive?"
> "Do you think that some of your body parts have dominance over others?"
> "Do you feel restricted in the way you use your body?"

Answers to these questions will direct clients' attention to the relationship between their movement patterns and patterns of general behaviour, as will the following suggestions:

> "By means of improvising, exaggerate* your dominant movement mode to the point where it turns into a burlesque. Amuse yourself by not only overstating the manner you favour, in terms of SPACE, TIME and ENERGY FLOW, but also exaggerate your preferred (habitual) postures, gestures, or any other body activities."
> "Improvise in a way that's unusual and strange to you."
> "Make yourself *uncomfortable,* and improvise in turn on what your discomfort gives rise to."
> "Do what you find difficult or even hate to do, in terms of body activities and movement elements. For instance, think about where you usually *are not* in SPACE, TIME, ENERGY FLOW."

---

*Exaggeration gives the feedback one receives from an experiment a greater impact.

"To experience the opposite extreme of your movement behaviour is vital to finding out what you are actually doing."

And in contrast to making yourself uncomfortable:

"Experiment now with a manner of movement you consider to be desirable, and *exaggerate that!*"

Discoveries made as a result of these strategies need to be checked out over a period of time. The way clients move in one particular session may merely reflect their "mood of the day."

comparing movement behaviour with day-to-day activities A very important question to put to clients at crucial stages of the therapy is *whether they think their behaviour in dance influences their behaviour in everyday life?*

After the client has completed a dance, some general questions might be:

review on completion of a dance "How do you feel in your body now?"
"Released?" "Frustrated?"
"Would you like to rest, or is there something else coming up that you would like to explore in movement?"
"What do you feel were your dance's most significant moments? Show me!"

The resulting dance could lead to:

"Which parts of that, if any, would you like to go over again? Which parts would you like to discard?"
"Is there any further dance statement you wish to make?"

Questions and answers will, of course, always be dealt with by a combination of movement and speech.

Lastly, a reference to *home practice* within the deductive approach:

examples for home practice The physical manifestations of the client's condition will become the basis for home practices. For example: in the case of the upper (thoracic) region being the culprit, home practice will focus on sensitising and mobilising the affected section as well as integrating its movement with the other parts of the spine. Similarly, feet and legs are often used merely to support the body or to move from place to place rather than taking an equal share in dance experimentations. In this latter case, sequences of foot and leg movements or "leg dances" *excluding the arms* will be suggested. Clients dominated perhaps by spatially direct movements with a sudden release of high energy would be advised to explore moving with a reduced amount of energy, and sustain the flow while moving, at least at times, along indirect pathways. These last two examples further illustrate the concept of *frames* (see p. 53).

Just as in the INDUCTIVE approach, home practice will always consist of physical tasks. Should psychical issues arise in the course of this, our advice to clients is not to try to deal with them at home, but bring them back to the therapist in the next session.*

c) INTERVENTION

Since we work within the orbit of movement our interventions are *motional* rather than verbal, although some verbal dialogue may accompany such action. We enter the movement situation of the client which enables us to *release, defuse* or *deflect* it *"from the inside."* This would result in working with a client on gradually transforming an excessively aggressive dance into a quieter mode. We see intervention as a kind of rescue operation. Other forms of working directly with the client we define as *interacting, teaching,* or *guiding.*

d) THE USE OF LANGUAGE

peripheral listening

In the INDUCTIVE and DEDUCTIVE approaches we have shown in a number of our strategies that asking the client suitable questions can help develop the dance material.

Frequently we may use speech as a backdrop or accompaniment to the dance; that is, the client continues to focus on the dance/movement experience, but at the same time attends to and takes in the therapist's spoken comments or suggestions. These will come organically and discreetly. It is left to the client to respond to or ignore

---

*For a vivid illustration of the DEDUCTIVE APPROACH and how it can alternate with INDUCTIVE episodes, see Chapter 5, "Denis' Journey."

them. (Clients will have been informed in advance of this particular strategy, accessible to them by what we call peripheral listening.)

use of movement words

There are a surprising number of words in our language which describe movement. Mettler (1969) has collated impressive lists of them which range from those describing subtle movement characteristics of the human face, to occurrences in the world around us (pp. 67–73). We have found that the use of words evocative of movement facilitates identification with motion.[10]

Sometimes words can be used to form *a link between thought and action.* Doing a movement while saying what it is: "meander," "quiver," "slink," "rise," may make the movement experience more concrete. Combining simple actions with appropriate words is another way of leading the reluctant or inexperienced client into dance. (See also The Role of Words in this chapter.) A client's exclamation or short statements accompanying an action are additional means of expression and may help to reduce self consciousness. But of course this would not apply in all cases.

There are also people who are very clever with words who tend to try to resolve only in their heads what has emerged from the "gut level." Putting gut level material into words is essentially reporting *from within the experience,* i.e. not interpreting or analysing it. Intellectualisation is not a reliable measure of true understanding.

What has come up from within cannot be adequately translated into words. Suzanne Langer (1953) describes how feelings are non-verbal experiences to which we can give no more than verbal labels. We have already referred to the avoidance of premature attempts to interpret feelings and insights in words in the Deductive Approach.

vocal communication

As well as the words themselves, the tone of voice used by the therapist plays an important part in the interaction with the client. Equally, its tempo and rhythm reflects the empathy the therapist has with the client's progress, communicating, for instance, encouragement, restraint or tranquility. Here, the sound of the therapist's voice takes on some aspects of the role of music.

e) THE USE OF MUSIC
The role of music and musical instruments as an accompaniment to dance is well known and has traditional and cultural connotations.

internal rhythms In dance as therapy, music has a special, reinforcing, facilitative role. However, the therapist needs to be sensitive about its use, since the client may be listening to an *inner music* which could be more eloquent and powerful than any other. It is important to recognize the possibility that any musical accompaniment may interfere with the authenticity of a dance, or with the purpose and quality of a given practice. We may all have experienced instances when music made us speed up to a degree which made us distort our movements or which cut across our mood when improvising and led us astray.

music as a background We have noticed that clients who gradually come into their own, detach themselves more and more from music, and prefer to follow their own internal dynamics. *Without music, we have no alternative other than to relate movements to ourselves.* [11] But as this presents considerable difficulties to clients in the early stages of therapy, we tend to support them with music which acts as no more than a *soundscape,* i.e. a musical "backdrop," providing an unobtrusive stimulus to dance experiences without being prescriptive. Even then clients must feel free to respond to the music if it suits them, or ignore it and follow their own impulse.

client's choice Then there is the music the client brings along to the session or chooses from what we offer. This chosen music will more than likely become readily integrated, and be supportive of his exploration. In many instances, such music will take the client deeper into himself and will gradually bring to consciousness important material to be worked on further in dance.

sharing music   In *group work,* too, we encourage members to bring to the session music which has a special meaning for them and to make suggestions about how they wish to use it. We give clients scope to dance to their music alone. As well, we invite others in the group to join in. This leads to a variety of responses which include, of course, further dance experiences for all the participants, and generally promotes group discussion. *Sharing music* for dance is another way for members of a group to get to know each other.

At the closing stages of a session, music makes an important contribution towards creating a calm atmosphere after a stormy improvisation, or to energising the client if his mood requires lifting. (We make sure we have a range of tapes at hand from which to choose appropriately.)

accompaniment *Percussion instruments,* which we often play as an accompaniment, provide an important stimulus to, as well as reinforcement of, the client's movement patterns: increasing their intensity, extending or shortening their duration, or suggesting repetition and variations.

Accompanying percussion with spoken comments can further illuminate and clarify the action. What may develop in one-to-one therapy is a *duet,* with the client-dancer and the therapist-musician alternating in taking the lead. Another variation on this interplay is for the two to change roles. Now the client becomes the musician. This creates a new situation with great therapeutic potential. The dancer-musician duet is also a useful experience for clients within the context of group sessions.

Some clients like to accompany themselves, either with percussive instruments or using simple body percussion, such as tapping or slapping. Sometimes they will chant or even sing. The sounds of the instrument, or of body tapping, or those produced by the voice, provide additional scope for working through emotional states and add pleasure to physical practices.

interplay   A percussive strategy we have used very successfully is for a client to be stationary, perhaps sitting in a chair. A partner, who could be the therapist, moves around holding a percussion instrument at every possible level, distance and direction, challenging the partner-client to reach it and make it sound. A further challenge for the stationary partner is to reach and strike the instrument with different parts of the body. Both these strategies provide great scope for variations and are particularly valuable for physically handicapped clients.

Distributing instruments at different places and at different levels in space provides further therapeutic possibilities. Clients can use this arrangement to choose whatever movements feel right, to reach a particular instrument. The next choice is how to play it and how long to stay with it before moving on. If a number of people are involved in this exploration, some interesting interplay of movement, sound and feelings will evolve.

The *sound qualities* of musical instruments depend to a large extent on the movement qualities which are applied to produce them. Hence the sound responses from the instruments reflect the wild, the gentle, tentative or agitated mood of the client playing them.

effects of instrument on player

Percussion playing is an invaluable means of letting off steam as well as of gaining control over the amount of energy we release with our actions.

The beauty of it is that you can beat a bongo as hard as you wish without hurting it, and gently stroke a tambour without it rejecting the intimacy.

And the *feedback of sound* from the instruments we play gives us the information we need to regulate our ENERGY FLOW *at will*. Regulating our ENERGY FLOW is important for dealing with people and situations comfortably and appropriately in everyday life.

f) THE USE OF IMAGES

the dynamic content of the image

The driving force in our work is *identification with motion*. For us it is not the visual aspect of an image, but its dynamics, its kinetic content, which we aim to internalise and transform into motion.

We would not, for instance, become the devil personified, but rather take into the body movements of devilishness which could be spiky, snakelike, aggressive or devious, slithering or pouncing.

Purely kinetic images are well suited for physiotherapeutic application; the tides for instance with their ebbing and flowing can be helpful in mobilizing a great many parts of the body. Such imagery promotes greater involvement and adds flavour and richness to the experience.

As well as adding *flavour* to a movement, which could even be expressed as tasting "delicious" or "disgusting," we may make use of associations with other sensory experiences. We can refer to a particular movement as making one "see red" (COLOUR), feel transparent (TEXTURE), or being spicy (SMELL).

dream images Dream images provide a rich source of material for exploration. Again it is with the dynamic aspect of the dreams that we identify for the purpose of interpretation. We would ask, for example:

> "How did the dream images move?"
> "Were they crawling?" "Flying?"
> "Do you think of them as aggressive or evasive?"

Interpreting these images physically in shape and motion leads to uncovering and understanding their significance. Images have to be brought into the here and now; "owning" them to the degree that occurs in dance may well open a door to a new phase in the therapy.

Feelings, which underlie the visual memories of a dream, may also be taken into the body quite readily. Many visual images carry an emotional meaning and are accompanied by a mood state, which itself may become the stimulus for a dance.

drawing images As well as dancing the dynamic content of images, the client can make drawings of them. To see facets of what has been going on inside depicted "out there," provides further ideas for developing the dance. If clients start out totally resistant to movement, one can first encourage them to draw or paint. This, a kinetic activity in itself, could lead eventually into dance.

It will be clear then that for us the crucial factor in the use of images is for them to be experienced in the body.

g) GROUP WORK

As stated in the Introduction, our method crystallised during the one-to-one study undertaken by Denis Kelynack and Johanna Exiner. Consequently, many of the examples we cite refer to the one-to-one situation. Nonetheless, we have found they can be adapted to and integrated with group work.

One of the major, if not the most important, reasons for group and partner work is to explore and expand ways of interaction with others.

breaking down large groups There are advantages in keeping groups small and reasonably homogeneous. However, where this is not possible, we form groups within groups or let members work with one another. In such instances it is very important that those who lead in a partnership be neither overconfident nor timid. Clear instructions on our part will prevent imbalances.

The more varied the problems are within a group, the harder it is to monitor and guide. For this reason we consider it essential for participants to have short one-to-one sessions with the therapist at agreed intervals, so that individual problems can be dealt with specifically.

partnering Facets of relating to one or more partners within the group can be experienced through sharing, exchanging, blending and contrasting movement qualities. Such interactions are initiated through "movement conversations" of action and reaction, question and answer, meeting and parting. In dancing together, group members will also become familiar with each others' physicality: differences in size, shape, level of energy, etc., to which they need to adjust. Throughout the progress of group work we provide assistance to partners who ask for or appear in need of help.

adjustment to
experience
Working with others brings a new experience to an individual's dance. This for some clients constitutes an enormous step. In such cases we allow time for gradual adjustment to acquaintance with the new and we are ready to accept withdrawal if the client feels too stressed. Though we invite clients to join the group and try to help their entry into it, we also respect those who clearly need a greater degree of solitude.

individual
needs
Group sessions obviously require a more general approach on the part of the therapist, yet we always base the content very directly on one or more clients' specific needs, such as to be better grounded, more flexible, slower and more organised, firm yet not tensed. Activities will be introduced to ensure that over a period of time each group member receives specific attention. It is part of the process to make group members aware that the procedure is of benefit to all. Everyone in the group learns what individual members need. And this in turn leads to better and deeper mutual understanding.

touch
In dance duets and in group work touch is intrinsic to the action of jointly creating shapes and movement patterns and in this context does not have personal connotations, important information for clients who are averse to, or who may actually be frightened of, physical contact. Interactions in dance therapy are symbolic. They should remain in the aesthetic domain as they do in all dance. For those clients who do find touch disagreeable, a strategy which has never failed, is to introduce simple movements back to back. Leaning against another without seeing the person is tolerable for most clients. In fact it surprises them that it is comfortable.

Whether a client partners the therapist or another client, it is *the dance* which forms the link between them. It is the dance which *connects* group members and at the same time *protects* from personal intrusions. The therapeutic focus rests on the way in which group members deal with a given *issue* in dance. If attraction or rejection does occur between group members, it can be dealt with by further work in dance, and ensuing discussion.

III. THE DANCE THERAPEUTIC RELATIONSHIP

The dance therapist acts as a catalyst between dance and the client. As the representative and facilitator of dance, he assists, supports, encourages, protects, teaches, intervenes. He guides and is guided by the client's needs and responds to them by means of dance. As we have said earlier, the dance therapist uses movements as readily as the verbal therapist uses words.

Interaction is based primarily on the therapist's capacity for *kinetic empathy,* that is, identifying with the client's physicality in shape and motion. Kinetic empathy is essential for the work to take place in the dance mode.

Although not always involving himself physically in the dance, the therapist is "with" the clients vicariously at all times. This affirms the clients' experience in the here and now, as well as giving the therapist a way of understanding what is going on, what is happening for the client. Being observed with empathy often provides the extra challenge that is needed for the work to be effective. This applies equally to physical and psychical conditions.

Frequently the client learns by means of example. For instance, the therapist may demonstrate how a particular movement such as an extension or a curve can be done to the full. However, it is important that the client's personal movement style is recognised and respected. Hence, the therapist makes every effort to transmit the *quality* of the movement, without for example attaching it to a distinctive sequence of gestures and thus avoids passing on his own idiosyncratic style.

The therapist is the recipient of the clients' dance; they dance to him as they would talk to him, they address him and want to be understood by him.

In the dance therapeutic relationship a *bridge is formed* by the dance. It connects and at the same time *leaves a space* which, though immeasurable, shields both therapist and client from becoming personally involved.

NOTES

1. *Body Activities*

   "Locomotion: Travelling along the floor as in walking, creeping, crawling, etc.
   Turning: Movements in which the body changes front
   Elevation: Taking off from the floor
   Falls: Movements which result in the major part of the body reaching floor level
   Gesture: Movements performed by the head, torso or limbs which do not necessarily involve any other *Body Activity* (These can be done from a variety of stances, e.g. standing, sitting, kneeling, lying etc.)"
   (from Exiner and Lloyd 1973, p. 12)

2. In a series of films entitled *Dance As An Art Form*, produced by Chimera Prods., N.Y. 1973, Murray Louis defines the elements of dance as SHAPE, SPACE, TIME & MOTION. We deduce from the way he interprets MOTION in dance that ENERGY FLOW is what *he* means also.

3. The authors' modification of Laban's Eight Effort Actions:

	SPACE	*TIME*	*ENERGY FLOW*
Punch:	direct	sudden	high-free
Slash:	indirect	sudden	high-free
Press:	direct	sustained	high-bound
Wring:	indirect	sustained	high-bound
Dab:	direct	sudden	low-bound
Flick:	indirect	sudden	low-bound
Glide:	direct	sustained	low-free
Float:	indirect	sustained	low-free

4. Movement modes are reflective of either the client's true personality or of an adopted *persona*. Persona (Latin for "theatrical mask") is a Jungian term standing for the way in which a person chooses to present himself to the world.

5. *Induction* is the process of inferring a general law or principle from the observation of particular instances.

   Deduction is inferring by reasoning from generals to particulars.

6. Individual dance therapists will draw on their knowledge and expertise in techniques such as the Bartenieff Fundamentals, Feldenkrais, Alexander and various forms of Yoga.

   Exercises from the techniques of dance masters Lester Horton, Erick Hawkins and Murray Louis have also proved useful.
   We believe in familiarising ourselves with as many movement-dance techniques as possible since different styles suit different clients.

7. Disharmonies of this nature may be due to genetic factors or to a previous or

current physical injury, psychical trauma, an environmental or social or yet other circumstance which the client is exposed to.

Invariably some of the causes are in a way interactive.

8. When faced with what appear to be complex physical conditions, we will of course work in consultation with a physiotherapist.

9. In the film *Why Man Creates* (made by Soul Bass & Associates U.S.A. 1969) the exploratory stage of the creative process is considered to be a journey of discovery. It is a kind of *playing* with the given material, *a fooling around.* "When you get something worth saving, worth using," says the commentary, "that is when the game stops and the work begins." By paying attention to such signals one adds purpose to the spontaneity of a dance improvisation whether in an artistic or therapeutic milieu.

10. Guidelines for achieving these aims can be found in *Teaching Creative Movement,* Exiner & Lloyd, Angus & Robertson 1973.

11. This statement was first made by Dr. John Lloyd when observing dance therapy sessions.

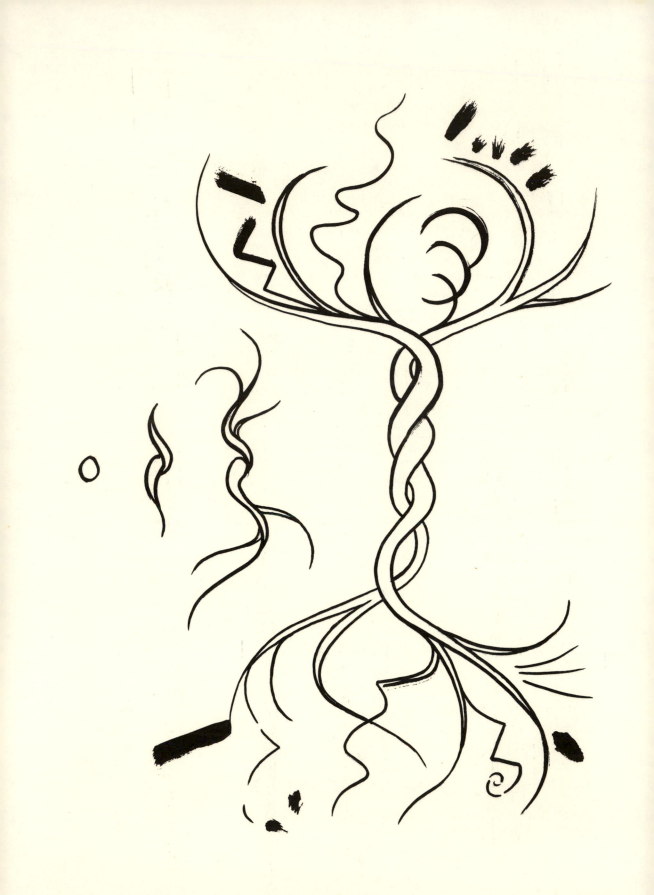

Chapter 5

DENIS' JOURNEY—A DANCE THERAPEUTIC EXPERIENCE

*"You are not the same people that left that station
Or who will arrive at any terminus."*

T. S. Eliot: *Four Quartets* III

Being a counselling psychologist has meant working with clients using verbal communication. I found my first introduction to non-verbal ways of working a revelation. My introduction to body work came when it was recommended that as part of my training as a group counsellor I go to a master class conducted by Will Schutz.

I took part in Will's one-week residential course in New England, N.S.W., in 1971. A trained Rolfer* and also a talented therapist, he demonstrated for the group the way in which Rolfing brings to the surface traumata and conflicts acquired in childhood, and showed us ways of processing them while simultaneously working on the deep muscle. He trained us in what he called "body reading" which was a diagnostic reading of holding patterns in the body's deep musculature. To the trained eye such reading would in his view be indicative of inhibitions and neurotic patterns of responding to the world.

In the same year I attended a Dance Therapy Workshop given by Tamara Greenberg of the Center for Energetic Studies in Berkeley, California, and I was also finding out about the work of Moshe Feldenkrais. I followed up this experience with a visit to Esalen Institute (Big Sur), where I was able to begin my own course of Rolfing and I also learnt about the work of Anna Halprin, the doyenne of healing dance at that time. Her workshops used the natural environment as a setting for dance/

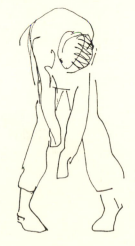

---

*Dr. Ida Rolf created this concept of deep tissue massage which changes posture by releasing long held tensions in the muscle fascia.

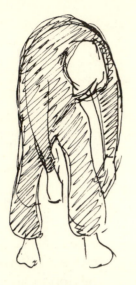

movement and also made extensive use of drawings ("visualisations"). She made use of African drums as a stimulus for expressive movement and encouraged dancers to get in touch with their primitive or basic aspects.

My interest in the depth and power in therapies which involved a recognition of the body in movement, action techniques as they are sometimes called, carried me through to a more detailed study of dance in the Graduate Diploma in Movement and Dance at the Institute of Early Childhood Development in Melbourne.

This course broadened my experience of dance itself and introduced me to the work of Rudolf Laban.

These influences, together with my long-time passion for the visual and performing arts, drew me towards the study of dance as therapy. I began teaching the Psychology and Dance component of the Movement and Dance Graduate Diploma and moved on to lecture in the Graduate Certificate of Dance Therapy course, in which Hanny* Exiner was also involved. My particular area concerned the nature of the therapeutic relationship and Hanny's was in the area of dance. We realised that in order to achieve a greater synthesis of our material we should collaborate. Thus came our mutual decision to work together.

Once Hanny and I began working we both took on *two* special roles for the purposes of our research:

client-colleague, and
therapist-colleague,

since we were not only taking the roles of client and therapist but also reviewing and assessing the process as we went along. The role of client was for me the most effective way of learning. I became the case we were studying and I also discussed the case with Hanny as co-worker.

The issues which I began exploring were of two sorts: firstly, day-to-day problems which presented themselves as part of my everyday existence and secondly, large issues concerning my long-term goals and values, my "quest" or life's journey and my sense of the meaning of life itself.

My goals were that I wanted to be more focussed, more direct in my

---

*short for Johanna.

dealings with people. I wanted to be able to go straight to any given objective. And I wanted also to rediscover a sense of childish delight and fun which I felt I'd lost. And as I have said, a long-term goal was concerned with finding a spiritual path.

There were also issues to do with my *persona*. I disliked some of the inbuilt characteristics which had been with me since childhood, my desire to please and ingratiate myself with others, my "niceness," my inability, as I saw it, to stand up for what I believed in; in other words, my lack of "iron in the soul." These aspects of myself had been the subject of earlier therapy sessions but never tried out and dealt with as completely as they were in dance. I was aware that these issues implied concerns about my expressive style: the masculine and feminine aspects, spontaneity and control, seriousness versus playfulness, body image and its connection with my use of the kinesphere, the relationship between my inner and outer worlds. At that time I had a pituitary tumour which was surgically removed and which needed further radiotherapy. I was reluctant to undergo this post-operative therapy as I knew of its unpleasant side effects. I also feared the aftermath of the loss of my pituitary gland which I had thought might mean a drop in energy and my overall capacity.

From the outset the focus of our work was the body. The early work with this emphasis encouraged me to feel each movement in the whole body. The fuller sensing of the body began with the feet and ankles since I knew that I needed to come down in my body awareness from the *centre of levity* to the *centre of gravity,* in other words to feel my connection with the earth.

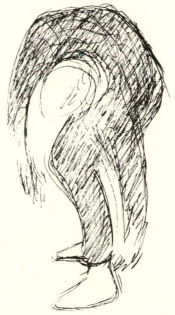

Our early sessions were concerned with my attempts to move in a way which expressed strength and power, and at the same time, openness and preparedness. This also meant work on the upper body; breathing into the upper area of the rib cage, mobilising the sternum and expanding the upper chest to arrive at a more upright posture. The change in posture, combined with a greater capacity to turn without losing balance (enhanced by work on feet and ankles in home practice) enabled me to move in a more flexible and yet strong dance.

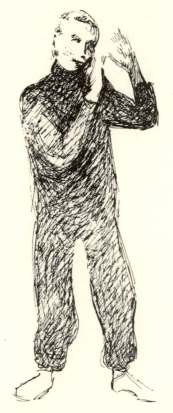

Also in the early sessions it was important for me to stand up for myself against imagined enemies. For instance, in one session I was practising strengthening exercises for my feet and ankles at the bar in front of a mirror, and at the same time I was reporting to Hanny my observations. I noticed that my knees tended to collapse together, and this seemed to me like a display of weakness. It became obvious to me that my habitual way of walking and holding the body had produced a shortening of tendons and unless these tendons were lengthened I would find it hard to overcome this "weakness." This brought up something of significance to me and led to an exploration of my father's walk, and in dance to a further experiencing of the sense of the introjected father. The dance revealed to me the extent to which I was still carrying ambivalent feelings about my father and my identification with him.

In a much later session I worked more deeply still by "becoming the issue" in dance. I began by continuing my confrontation of nameless forces, or enemies, and it was not until Hanny confronted me with her comment that I was still avoiding dealing with the issues in dance, and suggested that I take them into the body and allow them to be expressed through me rather than as outside entities, that I realised that what came through in the resulting dance was a dance of an archetypal father figure or tribal elder. This brought up for me the all-important issues of my response to others and my willingness to take on those responsibilities in full.

Learning a fuller sensing of the body in movement gave me more control of my movements. I practised stopping, turning, rising and falling. I found myself daring to be my full height, while I also felt myself firmly rooted to the ground. My posture changed and I began to feel more in control of *events* in my life as well as in my body. At the same time I felt a changed response in the people with whom I was in contact. They responded more positively and with deeper respect for my wishes.

This changed balance was not easy to adapt to. I realised how much investment I had had in previous attitudes (like not wanting to take my full rights and responsibilities). So the changes in my relationships, a direct result of my change in attitude, carried with them some broader insights. These changes were the outcome of my increased capacity to take control of my movements and to fill the space I actually do occupy.

At the beginning of each session Hanny would inquire how I was and, in response, I would usually indicate where in my body I felt a discomfort. Hanny's questions sometimes focussed this awareness more closely on a specific awareness of a body part, e.g. "Is there a part of your body that needs attention, that feels neglected?" etc. In the act of acknowledging this I found I was already moving that part and preparing to warm-up the body with that part as starting point. If I did not go further into a warm-up on my own, Hanny would suggest that I show her in what way my discomfort *resonated in my whole body.* Sometimes she might say simply: "Can you dance about it?" In the early part of each session she did not address herself directly to any problem as such, but rather sought to gain an impression of what was happening in the body and what it needed. Her response to my initial expression of the problem was kinesthetic.

From this initial phase a warm-up developed which was based on presenting problems as they were expressed in the body. In this phase Hanny might actively assist me to mobilise a body part by adjusting my posture or by using imagery, e.g. "Try directing your sternum towards the light."

As the work progressed a form emerged which allowed for a succession of dance statements, each one a development of its predecessor. In any one session there could be two, three, or even four successive dance statements, after the initial warm-up. To facilitate this progress Hanny might extend the warm-up to enable me to reach a fuller more complete dance/movement.

My work on strength, power, flexibility and readiness to fight formed a basis for a further stage along the therapeutic path. (I use the word therapeutic here to denote "growth and change".) At times the metaphorical path became the subject of my dance. I would find myself treading a path which seemed to symbolise my journey. The way in which I trod this path came to represent my own, idiosyncratic way of moving through life. The knowledge that I could choose to walk this path in a way I thought of as desirable, and that I could leave behind or abandon earlier

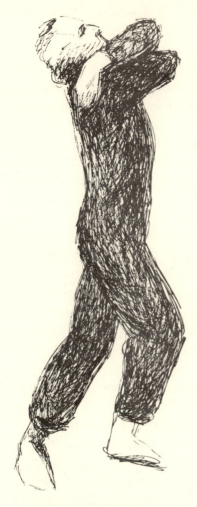

ways of moving, discarding old habits and taking on new ones, and that this could be done in dance, was enormously reassuring to me. Increasing one's repertoire of behaviour and response is part of growth and change, we know, but integrating the new patterns into one's daily life requires practice and reinforcement.

This reinforcement came in part from acquaintances who responded more positively to me (without commenting on any noticeable changes in me) and in part from Hanny (who *did* see the changes in my dance and in my body).

Eventually after two years of work, the moment arrived when I could move further along this path than I could ever have contemplated at the beginning. This happened in a session in which I had started to use vocal sounds in conjunction with movement and which repeated my familiar pattern of confrontation of outside forces. Hanny asked me if I knew the identity or nature of these entities. I replied that I had no idea of who or what they were. At this point Hanny (again) suggested that I "become them," that I allow them to be part of me instead of outside me, and hence alien to my experience. I responded and what emerged was a dance of gentle, compassionate, protective fatherliness. I had moved on from the struggle to become myself and *not* my real father, to becoming the essential Father. The meaning of this for me was in terms of a sense of responsibility for others, something I had not felt I was worthy to assume.

The dance theme was a slow walk with arms outstretched, hands extended in a gesture of protection and blessing. Its simplicity and power was very moving and allowed me to understand the inhibitions I had been feeling up to this time to allowing the fullest expression of "fatherliness" and the desire to nurture others. This work was the culmination of a consistent and systematic exploration of all I had brought to the early sessions: a synthesis of seemingly disparate issues.

As the work developed still further it deepened and came to have more complex, more far-reaching meanings than it had initially. The work in dance enabled a wide-ranging exploration of different modes of expression in themes which included for instance the lighter, more playful and spontaneous ways of being, as well as ironic, "distancing" attitudes. I found that the dance would take me more deeply into the feeling, and further, that through the dance the feeling would develop and change.

This kind of transformation of feeling, accompanied by insights about its significance in my everyday life, became more and more a familiar process to me, and I was able to trust the process to the extent that I opened myself up to the possibility of a full and free identification with the fatherly aspects of my own father, and through this, with my own role as a father figure.

The power of dance to heal and restore a person who is in a state of imbalance in a physical sense was illustrated by three particularly important episodes in our research. During my radiotherapy, a period of three weeks only, but with side-effects lasting for a month afterwards, I came to the sessions with physical problems: nausea, bowel upsets, low energy, headaches, etc.

In the first of these I complained of a heaviness. It felt like a burden and I placed it above my head. Hanny suggested I show her the extent of the burden, its actual dimensions, by any means I liked. I outlined it with upstretched hands. I moved it to left and right, rocking the head. Then I felt I could take it onto my left shoulder. It really felt as though I had moved it, but I could do no more with it. I wasn't sure where to go with it. Then Hanny suggested I could take the burden further into the body if I wished. It then moved to cover the trunk, arms and head. I felt it constricted me by its weight, but I could move it nonetheless. Then I compared it to a chain mail garment. I moved in space and used arm gestures, but slowly. Suddenly I felt that the garment had a positive side, it actually protected me and the sense of its burdensomeness disappeared. I welcomed it.

I came to the next session feeling nauseous and dyspeptic. I complained of a "tremulous" feeling in the upper body, especially in the solar plexus. With Hanny's encouragement I mobilised the scapulae, the sternum, the shoulders and eventually the whole of the back, neck and shoulder area.

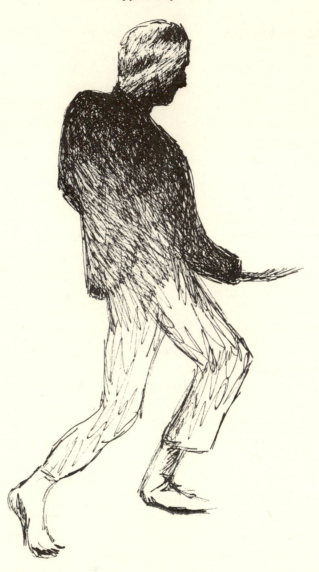

The movement quality I first wanted was tightly controlled and "held" (bound flow). I was holding on to the tension while carefully mobilising the various parts of the upper body.

To help me loosen up Hanny asked me to "indulge" in the movement. Then she asked where the feeling "was not," and we discussed the possibility of moving the feeling into the legs and feet. To help me differentiate the parts of the back I was trying to mobilise, Hanny used a hands-on technique: gently moving the shoulder to allow me to release it. This permitted a more open and fuller movement statement so that although the ensuing dances still focussed on the upper body, the movements had become more expansive and used up more of the kinesphere. I began to use different levels and eventually worked from the floor, moving the spine in convulsive undulations.

The effect of this dance was to disperse the "tremulous" (anxious) feeling and invigorate the body. I remained somewhat debilitated due to the aftermath of the ray treatment, but I had regained something of my sense of my whole body, my completeness and wholeness as a person.

To the next session I brought the plastic mask that had been made by the radiotherapy team to ensure that my head remained firmly in position during the treatments. I told Hanny I hated the mask, representing as it did the impersonality of machine therapy. I held the mask and looked at it and further associations came: I realised how much fear I had had of the possible bad side-effects of the treatment and at the same time that the mask reminded me of death.

I threw the mask away, saying "I don't want to keep it. It's come to represent something demonic." Hanny suggested that I take my sense of revulsion into the body. What ensued was a dance of exorcism to the accompaniment of Hanny's drum (which she managed to make sound like a didgeridoo*). The dance began with a smoothing movement of the hands on the head; taking the toxins from the head and flinging them away with strong flicking movements. The dance developed into broader gestures, reaching out to the front and scooping or gathering some healing substance from the air. It became increasingly stylised and formal, a ritualistic casting out of toxins, ending in an open standing posture with arms outstretched.

At the time I felt I had achieved a real sense of delivery from the aftermath of the radiotherapy and of my negative feelings about it. This was an important part of my recovery. I could begin the process of physical recovery freed from the encumbrance of my resentment at having had to have it at all, my superstitions in effect.

Reviewing the session on videotape months later, I saw how the dance had developed and changed from an expression of pain, fear and loathing, into a calm, assured, serene assertion of my power to help myself.

The self-healing process had begun in dance.

---

*didgeridoo: an Australian aboriginal wind instrument.

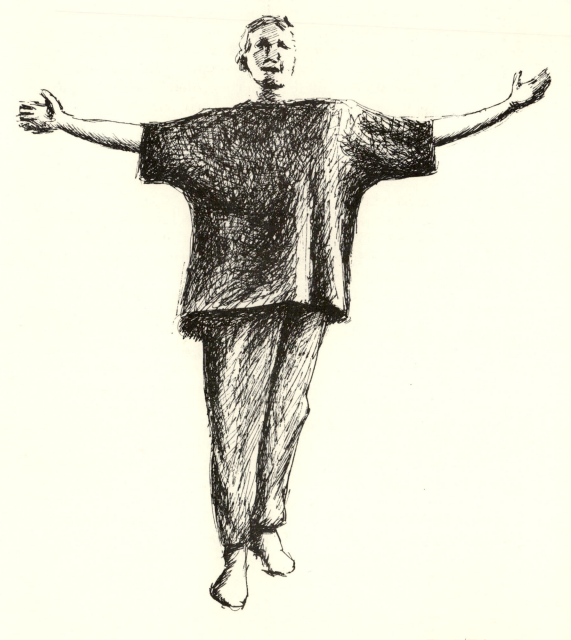

Denis Kelynack

APPENDICES

Appendix 1

PROPRIOCEPTION

Paired with the kinesthetic sense is the labyrinthine sense or sense of balance. Its location is in the labyrinth, the intricate structure of the inner ear. The section which holds the mechanism for attaining balance is the vestibule. It is filled with fluid substances and contains small bonelike particles. When movement occurs these particles called otoliths act upon the receptors, these being hair cells which then conduct the stimuli to the brain. Stimulation occurs not so much through movement as such, but through *"changes in rate or direction of movement"* (Telford and Sawrey, 1968, p. 120) as well as through changes in gravitational forces. "The receptors involved in kinesthetic sense and in the sense of balance, or the labyrinthine sense, are grouped together as proprioceptors. The two senses are alike in that they are both stimulated by the action of the body itself" (p. 118).

Also very closely related to the kinesthetic sense is the tactile sense or sense of touch. Practical evidence for this can be gained through making oneself aware of the increase in intensity while experiencing a gliding motion of the hand over a surface, swishing one's feet through leaves or even walking in the wind. When dancing, movements feel more vital and alive if space is considered a tangible substance and the ground a surface to work WITH rather than just a base which supports the body. Physiological evidence for interaction between touch and movement is given in *Psychology* by Stagner and Karwoski (New York, McGraw Hill, 1952): "While the kinesthetic impulses travel up the spinal cord in a tract separate from the skin-senses . . . the two sets of impulses are united in the cortex. This is functionally necessary because touch and muscle sense co-operate so closely in guiding motor adjustment to the body" (p. 149).

Appendix 2

THE CHOREOGRAPHIC PROCESS

Helmi Vent and Helma Drefke describe the choreographic process in the context of dance for schools in their book *Gymnastik/Tanz,* published by Cornelsen Schwann, Düsseldorf, 1988 (translated by J. Exiner).

The first few paragraphs of this section deal with the re-creation of other choreographers' work not relevant to dance therapy. However, what they call the "second path" is highly relevant to our work. They say it "leads, via improvisation, as a means of exploration and 'spontaneous forming' to composition. In detail this means:

> *playful searching, experimenting,* collecting of experiences and impressions with/through various possibilities of action and expression in movement

> *finding (out), inventing* and *'retaining'* committing to memory of movement forms, motives and short sequences

> *repeating, practising,* in certain circumstances improving of movement forms discovered through exploration/improvisation. This practice of movement patterns and sequences found on one's own is a form of reproduction within the process of production, during which improvised and reproduced segments alternate, interweave and complement one another

> *varying* and *combining* of the found and selected movement motives and themes

> *composing/forming* of the processed movement material with intentional consideration of compositional criteria

> *reproducing, repeating, reinforcing* of one's own movement composition

under certain circumstances renewed *revision, alteration,* re-shaping of the study."

Vent and Drefke conclude this section as follows: "In both of the mentioned paths [recreation and creation] the discrete phases of forming should be supplemented repeatedly by means of mutual observation, reflection and discussion, e.g. about the given or the (self) created (movement) material, about possible structures, planning and the aim of the composition under review, about difficulties and obstacles in the process of formation, about possibilities of change and of improvement. That means that phases of reflection and mutual discussion should alternate repeatedly with phases of search, exploration, discovery, retention, repetition, practice, alteration and integration" (pp. 135/6).

Appendix 3

BODY IMAGE

Schilder* in his classic book *The Image and Appearance of the Body*† describes body image as "the picture of our own body which we form in our mind, that is to say the way in which the body appears to ourselves" (p. 11). He considers it as being a composite of the way we experience ourselves physically, the way we perceive ourselves conceptually and the impression we have formed of what our body looks like. More often than not we are at loggerheads with the picture we have of our bodies; we want to see ourselves as different to what we actually are. Instead of actively working on changing ourselves, Schilder refers to attempted transformations by means of clothing and decorations such as jewellery. He cites a number of healthier ways of changing, amongst them gymnastics and, very specifically, dance. He believes that dance is by its very nature "a method of changing the body-image and loosening its rigid shape" (p. 208).

---

*Paul Schilder, M.D., Ph.D., Research Professor of Psychiatry, New York University

†International Universities Press Inc., New York, 1950.

Appendix 4

TWO STATEMENTS ON DANCE THERAPY

Excerpt from a press release* under the heading of "Dance Therapy: Dance is the best medicine" which corresponds closely with our view discussed in "Observation and Appraisal" (Chapter 4):

> "Thinking and feeling are expressed in the soundless yet very audible language of the body, tensions and contortions of the psyche become visible through it. The personality of a person becomes apparent in his physical appearance, posture and movement pattern. Dance therapy uses these expressions of the body as a diagnostic tool and as a therapeutic method. With its help we can ascertain how a person is psychically structured and where his strengths and weaknesses lie. And on this basis the movement repertoire of the client will be addressed, leading to changes in his movement mode and to an expansion of his movement vocabulary."

As to dance therapy in general, the philosophy of the Langen Institute's approach is very much in sympathy with our own:

> "All dance therapeutic methods share the use of dance and movement as *primary* [italics added] tools of change. Dance therapy is based on the psycho physical unity of Man; this means that the personality of a client is also shown in his physical appearance, his posture and his movement pattern. Dance therapy as a holistic method integrates different therapeutic approaches. E.g. you can improve the body movement technique with stroke patients and other invalids and increase their body awareness.
> Dance therapy always aims at the expansion of a client's scope for experience and development in the emotional, cognitive and physical domains."†

---

*Issued by the Langen Institute, Director: Wally Kaechele, and the Bundesverband Für Tanztherapie, Hofstrasse 16, Marienburg, 4019 Monheim, Germany

†The above statements have been selected and translated by the authors.

GLOSSARY

catharsis: from the Greek *katharsis* a cleansing, used here as a shedding of damaging psycho-physical constraints

mode: from the Latin *modus* meaning "measure" or "manner"

style: manner of creative, artistic expression. Derived from the Latin *stylus*, a writing implement. It became a metaphor for how something was written rather than the content of the writing

transcendent: going beyond one's ordinary limits

transformation: change in nature, form and awareness, metamorphosis

Glossary of Medical Terms

"Central Nervous System (CNS), one of the two main divisions of the nervous system of the body, consisting of the brain and the spinal cord. The central nervous system processes information to and from the peripheral nervous system and is the main network of coordination and control for the entire body. The brain controls many functions and sensations, as sleep, sexual activity, muscular movement, hunger, thirst, memory, and the emotions. The spinal cord extends various types of nerve fibers from the brain and acts as a switching and relay terminal for the peripheral nervous system.

"The brain and spinal cord are composed of gray matter and white matter. The gray matter contains primarily nerve cells and associated processes; the white matter consists of bundles of predominantly myelinated nerve fibers. The central nervous system develops from the embryonic neural tube, which first appears as the neural fold in the third week of pregnancy. The cavity of the neural tube is retained after birth in the ventricles of the brain and in the central canal of the spinal cord" (pp. 207–208)

"Endocrine System, the network of ductless glands and other structures that elaborate and secrete hormones directly into the bloodstream, affecting the function of specific target organs. Glands of the endocrine system include the thyroid and the parathyroid, the anterior pituitary, the posterior pituitary, the pancreas, the suprarenal glands and the gonads. The pineal gland is also considered an endocrine gland because it is ductless, although its precise endocrine function is not established.

"The thymus gland, once considered an endocrine gland, is now classified in the lymphatic system. Various other organs have some endocrinologic function. Secretions from the endocrine glands affect various processes throughout the body, as metabolism, growth, and secretions from other organs" (p. 395).

"Immune System, a biochemical complex that protects the body against pathogenic organisms and other foreign bodies. The system incorporates the humoral immune response (humoral: relating to body fluids as distinct from cells), which produces antibodies to react with specific antigens, and the cell-mediated response, which uses T cells to mobilize tissue macrophages in the presence of a foreign body. The immune system also protects the body from invasion by creating local barriers and inflammation. The local barriers provide chemical and mechanic defenses through the skin, the mucous membranes, and the conjunctiva. Inflammation draws polymorphonuclear leucocytes and neutrophils to the site of the injury where these phagocytes engulf the invading organism. The humoral response and the cell-mediated response develop if these first-line defenses fail or are inadequate to protect the body. The humoral immune response is especially effective against bacterial and viral invasion and employs B cells that produce appropriate antibodies. The principal organs of the immune response system include the bone marrow, the thymus, and the lymphoid tissues. The system also employs peripheral organs, as the lymph nodes, the spleen, and the lymphatic vessels. The antigen-antibody reactions of the immune system activate the complement system, which removes antigens from the body. The complement system contains several discrete proteins that function to produce lysis of the antigenic cells. The humoral response may begin immediately on invasion by the antigen or may start as long as 48 hours later." (p. 571)

Note. All the above definitions are excerpts from Mosby's *Medical & Nursing Dictionary* 2nd Edition (ed. Nancy L. Mullins). The C.V. Mosby Company, St. Louis, Missouri, USA, 1986. Reprinted by permission.

BIBLIOGRAPHY AND WIDER READING

BIBLIOGRAPHY

Berne, E.M.D., *Beyond Games and Scripts.* Ballantine Books, New York, 1976.

Boas, F., "Origins of Dance" in *Dance Therapy: Roots and Extensions.* Proceedings of the Sixth Annual Conference of the American Dance Therapy Association. ADTA, Columbia, Maryland, 1972.

Bodenwieser, G., *The New Dance.* Published posthumously by Marie and Eric Cuckson, Sydney, 1970.

Buckley, V., *Poetry and Morality.* Chatto and Windus, London, 1959.

Bunge, M., *The Mind-Body Problem. A Psychobiological Approach.* Pergamon Press, Oxford, 1980.

Burnshaw, Stanley, *The Seamless Web: Language—Thinking, Creature—Knowledge, Art—Experience.* George Braziller Inc., New York, 1970. Also published in paperback by George Braziller Inc., New York, 1991 with an introduction by John Dickey.

Camara, E.G., Danao, T.C., "The Brain and the Immune System—a Psychosomatic Network" in *Psychosomatics* 30, 1989.

Campbell, J., *Myths to Live By.* Phantom Books, N.Y. 1988.

Dunn, A.J., "Psychoneuroimmunology for the Psychoneuroendocrinologist: a Review of Animal Studies of Nervous System-Immune Interactions" in *Psychoneuro-indocrinology* 14/4, 1989.

Dunn, A.J., "Recent Advances in Psychoneuroimmunology" in *Current Opinion in Psychiatry.* Vol. 3 1990 No. 1.

Espenak, L., *Dance Therapy, Theory and Application.* Charles Thomas, Springfield, Ill., 1981.

Exiner, J. and Lloyd, P., *Teaching Creative Movement.* Angus and Robertson, Sydney, 1973.

Gardner, H., *Frames of Mind. The Theory of Multiple Intelligences.* Basic Books Inc., New York, 1983.

Gelb, M., *Body Learning.* Aurum Press, London, 1981.

H'Doubler, M.N., *Dance: a Creative Art Experience.* University of Wisconsin Press, 1966.

Hollingdale, R.J., *Nietzsche.* Routledge and Kegan Paul, London, Boston, 1973.

Koestler, A., *The Act of Creation.* Hutchinson & Co., London, 1964.

Laban, R., *The Mastery of Movement.* Macdonald and Evans, London, 1960.

Lange, R., *The Nature of Dance.* MacDonald, London, 1975.

Langer, S.K., "The Cultural Importance of the Arts" in *Aesthetics and Problems of Education.* R.A. Smith (ed.). Illinois Press, Urbana, New York, Tokyo, 1971.

Langer, S.K., *Feeling and Form: A Theory of Art.* Scribner, New York, 1953.

Maisel, E. (ed.), *The Alexander Technique.* Thames and Hudson, London, 1974.

Martin, J., *Introduction to the Dance.* Dance Horizon Inc., N.Y. 1965.

May, R., *Love and Will.* Dell Pub. Co., New York, 1969.

Mettler, B., *Ten Articles on Dance.* Mettler Studios, Tucson, Arizona, undated.

Mettler, B., *Materials of Dance as a creative art activity.* Mettler Studios, Tucson, Arizona, 1960.

Mullins, N.L., (ed.) *Mosby's Medical & Nursing Dictionary* 2nd Edition. The CV Mosby Company, St. Louis, Missouri, 1986.

Öhman, R., Freeman, H.L., Franck Holmkvist, A., Nielzén, S. (eds), *Interaction between Mental and Physical Illness. Needed Areas of Research.* Springer-Verlag, Berlin, Heidelberg, New York, London, Paris, Tokyo, 1989.

Pentony, P., *Models of Influence in Psychotherapy.* Free Press, New York, 1981.

Peter-Bolaender, M., *Tanz und Imagination.* Junfermann, Paderborn, 1992.

Pierce, A. and Pierce, R., *Expressive Movement. Posture and Action in Daily Life, Sport and the Performing Arts.* The Center of Balance, Redlands, Cal., 1989.

Popper, K.R. and Eccles, J.C., *The Self and its Brain. An Argument for Interactionism.* Springer International, 1977.

Rickman, J. (ed.) General Selection from the Works of Sigmund Freud. The Hogarth Press and the Institute of Psychoanalysis, London, 1953.

Rieder, H., *Sportwissenschaftliches Lexikon* quoted in *Tanzen.* Deutscher Bundesverband Tanz, Georg Kallmeyer Verlag, 3/89.

Sacks, O., *A Leg To Stand On.* Pan Books, London, 1986.

Saphier, D., "Neurophysiological and Endocrine Consequences of Immune Activity" in *Psychoneuroendocrinology* Vol. 14, No. 1 & 2, 1989.

Schilder, P., *The Image and Appearance of The Body.* International Universities Press, New York, 1950.

Stagner, R. and Karwoski, T.F., *Psychology.* McGraw Hill, New York, 1952.

Telford, C.W. and Sawrey, J.M., *Psychology.* Brooks/Cole Publishing Company, Belmont, Cal., 1968.

Vent, H. and Drefke, H., *Gymnastik/Tanz.* Cornelsen Schwann, Düsseldorf, 1988.

Watzlawick, P., Weakland, C.E., Fisch, R., *Change.* Norton & Co., New York, London, 1974.

Whitehouse, M., "Reflections on a Metamorphosis" in *Impulse,* 1969/70, (Extensions of Dance) Impulse Publications Inc., San Francisco, Cal.

Wolman, B., *Psychosomatic Disorders.* Plenum Publishing Co., New York, 1988.

Yukic, T.S., *Fundamentals of Recreation.* Harper & Row, New York, London, 1970.

WIDER READING

SCIENCE/BODY MIND

Bergland, R., *The Fabric of Mind.* Penguin, Australia, 1985.

Camara, E.C. and Danao, T.C., "The Brain and the Immune System—A Psychosomatic Network." *Psychosomatics,* 30: 140–146, 1989.

Capra, F., *The Tao of Physics.* Shambhala Publications, Boston, Mass., 1991.

Capra, F., *Uncommon Wisdom, Conversations with Remarkable People.* Century Hutchinson Ltd., London, 1987.

Capra, F., *The Turning Point, Science, Society and the Rising Culture.* Flamingo, published by Fontana Paperbacks, London, 1983.

Chopra, D., *Quantum Healing. Exploring the Frontiers of Mind/Body Medicine.* Bantam Books, New York, 1989.

Feldenkrais, M., *Awareness Through Movement.* Harper Row, New York, 1971.

Fitt, S., *Dance Kinesiology.* Schirmer Books, New York, 1988.

Furst, C., *Origin of the Mind—Mind Brain Connections.* Prentice-Hall, Englewood Cliffs, New Jersey, 1979.

Gould, S.J., *Ever Since Darwin. Reflections in Natural History.* Penguin Books, London, 1991 (first published by Burnell Books Ltd., 1978).

Green, S., *Physiological Psychology. An Introduction.* Routledge & Kegan Paul, London & New York, 1987.

Gregory, R.L., *Oxford Companion to the Mind.* Oxford University Press, Oxford, New York, 1987.

Jacob, F., *The Possible and the Actual.* Pantheon Books, New York, 1982.

Janner, L.D., Schwartz, E., Leigh, H., "The Relationship between Repressive and Defensive Coping Styles." *Psychosomatic Medicine,* 50:567–575, 1988.

Korneva, E.A., "Beginnings and Directions of Psycho Neuro Immunology." *International Journal of Psychophysiology* 25: 18–25, 1989.

Lamb, W., *Posture and Gesture. (An introduction to the study of physical behaviour).* G. Duckworth & Co. Ltd., London, 1965.

Lamb, W., *Body Code: The meaning of movement.* Routledge & Kegan Paul, London, 1979.

Lowen, A., *The Betrayal of the Body.* Collier, New York, 1967.

Oakley, D.A. (ed.), *Brain and Mind.* Methuen, New York, 1985.

Oakley, D.A. & Plotkin, H.C., *Brain, Behaviour & Evolution.* Methuen, New York, 1985.

Petzold, H. (ed.), *Leiblichkeit—philosophische, gesellschaftliche und therapeutische Perspektiven (Physicality—philosophical, social and therapeutic perspectives).* Junfermann Verlag, Paderborn, 1985.

Rappaport, B.S., "Carnal Knowledge. What the Wisdom of the Body has to Offer Psychotherapy." *Journal of Humanistic Psychology.* Vol. 15, No. 1. Winter 1975.

Springer, S.P. & Deutsch, G., *Left Brain, Right Brain.* Freeman, San Francisco, 1981.

Suzuki, D. and Hehner, B., *Looking at the Body.* Allen and Unwin, Sydney, 1989.

Thomas, L., *The Lives of a Cell.* Bantam Books, Inc., Toronto, New York, London, 1975.

Todd, M.E., *The Thinking Body.* Dance Horizons, New York, 1968.

Weisskopf, V.F., *Knowledge and Wonder. The Natural World as Man Knows It.* Anchor Books, Doubleday & Company Inc., Garden City, New York, 1966.

Zukav, G., *The Dancing Wu Li Masters. An Overview of the New Physics.* A Bantam Book published by arrangement with William Morrow & Company Inc., 1980.

DANCE

Bartal, L., Ne'Eman, N., *Movement Awareness and Creativity.* Souvenir Press Ltd., London, 1975.

Dell, C., *A Primer for Movement Description Using Effort-Shape and Supplementary Concepts.* Dance Notation Bureau, New York, 1970.

Duncan, I., *My Life.* Lowe & Brydone, London, 1968.

Exiner, J. & Lloyd, P., *Learning Through Dance.* Oxford Press, Melbourne, 1987.

Graham, M., *Blood Memory. An autobiography.* Doubleday, New York, 1991.

Graham, M., *The Notebooks of Martha Graham.* Harcourt Brace Jovanovich, New York, 1973.

Hanna, J.L., *To Dance is Human.* University of Texas, Austin, 1979.

Haselbach, B., *Improvisation, Dance, Movement.* Magnamusic-Baton, Stuttgart, 1976.

Hawkins, E., *The Body is a Clear Place.* A Dance Horizon Book, Princeton Book Company, Publishers. Princeton, N.J. 1992.

Kraus, R., *History of the Dance in Art and Education.* Prentice-Hall, New York, 1964.

Laban, R. & Lawrence, F.C., *Effort.* MacDonald & Evans, London, 1947.

Lange, R., *The Nature of Dance.* Macdonald & Evans Ltd., London, 1975.

Maletic, V., *Body, Space, Expressions.* Mouton de Gruyter, Berlin, 1987.

Martin, J., *The Modern Dance.* Dance Horizons, Brooklyn, 1965.

McFee, G., *Understanding Dance.* Routledge, New York, 1992.

Meerloo, J.M., *Dance Craze and Sacred Dance.* Peter Owen, London, 1962.

Murray, L., *Inside Dance.* St Martins Press, New York, 1980.

Nadel, M.H. & Nadel, C.C., *The Dance Experience.* Praeger, New York, 1970.

Preston-Dunlop, V. and Lahusen, S., *Schriftanz: A View of German Dance in the Weimar Republic.* Dance Books, London, 1990.

Redfern, B., *Dance, Art and Aesthetics.* Dance Books Ltd. of Cecil Court, London, 1983.

Russell, J., *Creative Dance in the Primary School.* Macdonald & Evans, London, 1965.

Shawn, T., *Every Little Movement.* Dance Horizon, New York, 1968.

Sheets-Johnstone, M., *The Phenomenology of Dance.* Dance Books Ltd., London, 1979 (first published 1966).

Spurgeon, D., *Dance Moves: from improvisation to dance.* Harcourt Brace Jovanovich, Sydney, 1990.

Thornton, S., *A Movement Perspective of Rudolf Laban.* Macdonald & Evans, London, 1971.

Ullman, L. (ed.), *Rudolf Laban Speaks about Movement and Dance.* Addlestone, Surrey, Laban Art of Movement Centre, 1971.

Wigman, M., *The Mary Wigman book: her writings edited and translated by Walter Sorell.* Wesleyan University Press, Middletown, Connecticut, 1975.

Wigman, M., *The Language of Dance.* Translated from the German by Walter Sorell, Wesleyan University Press, Middletown, Connecticut, 1966.

DANCE THERAPY

Adler, J., " 'Who is the Witness?' A description of authentic movement." *Contact Quarterly,* Winter 87.

Barlow, W., *The Alexander Principle. How to use your body.* Arrow Books Ltd., London, 1975.

Bartenieff, I. with Lewis, D., *Body Movement: Coping with the Environment.* Gordon & Breach, New York, 1980.

Bernstein, P.O. (ed.), *Eight Theoretical Approaches to Dance Therapy.* Kendall-Hunt, Dubuque, Iowa, 1979.

Bond, K., "Dance for children with dual sensory impairments." Thesis, La Trobe University, School of Ed. Teaching Centre, Melbourne, 1991.

Canner, N., *. . . And a Time to Dance.* Plays Inc., Boston, 1975.

Caplow-Lindner, E., Harpaz, L. and Samberg, S., *Therapeutic Dance/Movement. Expressive Activities for Older Adults.* Human Sciences Press, New York, 1979.

Chodorow, J., *Dance Therapy and Depth Psychology: the moving imagination.* Routledge, London, 1991.

Costonis, M.N. (ed.), *Therapy in Motion.* University of Illinois Press, Urbana, Chicago, London, 1978.

Dychtwald, K., *Body-Mind.* Third printing. A Jove Book, New York, 1981.

Fitt, S. & Riordan, A. (eds), *Focus on Dance IX: Dance for the Handicapped.* Journal of The American Alliance for Health, Physical Education, Recreation and Dance, Reston, Virginia 22091.

Guthrie, J. with Roydhouse, J., *Come and Join the Dance.* Hyland House, Melbourne, 1988.

Hörmann, K., *Durch Tanzen zum eigenen Selbst. Eine Einführung in die Tanz-therapie.* (*Through Dance to the Self. An introduction to dance therapy*) Goldmann Verlag, Munich, 1991.

Lerman, L., *Teaching Dance to Senior Adults.* Charles C Thomas Publisher, Springfield, Illinois, 1984.

Leventhal, M.B., "Healing through Rhythm and Movement." 10th Annual Body-Mind-Spirit Festival. London U.K. 1987.

Levy, F.J. (ed.), *Dance Movement Therapy. A Healing Art.* The American Alliance for Health, Physical Education, Recreation and Dance, Reston, Virginia, 1988.

Mason, K.C. (ed.), *Focus on Dance VII: Dance Therapy.* Journal of the American Alliance for Health, Physical Education, Recreation and Dance, Reston, Virginia 22091, 1974.

Mettler, B., "Creative Dance-Art or Therapy". (unpublished article). Tucson, Arizona, January, 1973.

Payne, H. (ed.), *Dance Movement Therapy. Theory and Practice.* Tavistock, Routledge, London, New York, 1992.

Petzold, H., *Integrative Bewegungs-und Leibtherapie. (Integrative Movement and Body Therapy).* Junfermann Verlag, Paderborn, 1989.

Salkin, J., *Body Ego Technique.* Charles C Thomas, Springfield, Ill., 1973.

Schoop, T., *Won't You Join The Dance.* Mayfield Pub. Co., Palo Alto (Calif.), 1974.

Smallwood, J.C., "Dance Therapy and the Transcendent Function." *American Journal of Dance Therapy,* 2 (1) (DT-3): 16–23.

Whitehouse, M., "Physical Movement and Personality." A talk given to the Analytical Psychology Club of L.A. in 1965. *Contact Quarterly,* Winter 87.

Wilke, E., Hölter, G., Petzold, H. (eds), *Tanztherapie – Theorie und Praxis. Ein Handbuch. (Dance Therapy – Theory and Practice. A Handbook.)* Junfermann Verlag, Paderborn, 1991.

PSYCHOLOGY

Bandler, R. and Grinder, J., *Frogs into Princes: Neurolinguistic programming.* Real People Press, Moab, Utah, 1979.

Bean, P. (ed.), *Mental Illness. Changes and Trends.* John Wiley & Sons, Chichester, 1983.

Borysenko, J., *Minding the Body, Mending the Mind.* Bantam Books, New York, 1987.

Erickson, M., *Uncommon Therapies.* Norton, New York, 1973.

Gardner, H., *Frames of Mind. The theory of multiple intelligence.* Basic Books Inc., New York, 1983.

Jung, C.G., *The Portable Jung.* Edited, with an introduction by Joseph Campbell. The Viking Press, New York, 1971.

Kellerman, S., *Your Body Speaks Its Mind.* Center Press, Berkeley, 1975.

Kellerman, S., *The Human Ground. Sexuality, Self and Survival.* Center Press, Berkeley, 1975.

Laing, R.D., *Wisdom, Madness and Folly.* MacMillan, London, 1985.

Masters, R., Houston, J. *Listening to the Body. The Psychological Way to Health and Awareness.* Delta Books, New York, 1978.

Miller, J. (ed.), *States of Mind. Conversations with Psychological Investigators.* British Broadcasting Corp., London, 1983.

Ornstein, R., *The Psychology of Consciousness.* Viking, New York, 1972.

Rogers, C.R., *A Way of Being.* Houghton Mifflin Co., Boston, 1980.

Stevens, J. O. (ed.), *Gestalt Is.* Real People Press, Utah, 1975.

Szasz, T., *The Myth of Mental Illness.* Paladin, London, 1972.

The Secret of the Golden Flower. A Chinese Book of Life. Translated and explained by Richard Wilhelm with a European Commentary by C.G. Jung. Routledge & Kegan Paul Ltd., London, 1931.

Watzlawick, P., *How Real is Real.* Vintage Books, New York, 1977.

Watzlawick, P. *The Situation is Hopeless but not Serious. (The Pursuit of Unhappiness)*. W.W. Norton, New York, 1983.

JOURNALS & PERIODICALS

ACHPER National Journal, Australian Council for Health, Physical Education, Recreation and Dance
American Journal of Dance Therapy
Conference Proceedings, American Dance Therapy Association, 1968–74.
Contact Quarterly
Dance Research Journal
Focus On Dance. American Alliance for Health, Physical Education and Recreation, Issue 7. 1974, entirely devoted to Dance Therapy.
Journal of Physical Education, Recreation and Dance (USA)
Musik-, Tanz- und Kunsttherapie. Zeitschrift für künstlerische Therapien, Georg Thieme Verlag, Stuttgart—New York.
Tanzen. Deutscher Bundesverlag Tanz e.V. Distribution through: "Ballett International" Verlags GmbH. Richard Wagner Strasse 33, Köln, Germany.
Tanz und Therapie. Journal of the Bundesverband für Tanztherapie e.V. Hofstrasse 16, Monheim, D 4019, Germany.

MISCELLANEOUS

Barta, F. & Geissman, M.G., *Die Beredsamkeit des Leibes. (The Eloquence of the Body)*. Residenz-Verlag, Salzburg/Wien, 1992.
Campbell, J., *The Hero With A Thousand Faces.* Paladin Grafton Books, London, 1988.
Campbell, J., *Myths To Live By.* The Viking Press, New York, 1972.
Feder, B. & Feder, E., *The Expressive Arts Therapies.* Prentice-Hall, Englewood Cliffs, New Jersey, 1981.
Hamel, P.M., *Through Music to the Self.* Shambala, Boulder, 1979.
Jersild, A.T., *When Teachers Face Themselves.* Bureau of Publications, Teachers College, Columbia University, 1955.
Jungmair, U.E., *Das Elementare Zur Musik- und Bewegungserziehung im Sinne Carl Orffs, Theorie und Praxis. (Primer for Music- and Movement Education in Carl Orff's sense, Theory and Practice.)* B. Schott's Sons, Mainz, 1992.
Lett, W. (ed.), *How the Arts Make a Difference in Therapy.* Papers from the Arts in Therapy Conference at La Trobe University, Melbourne, 1992. Australian Dance Council (Victoria), Ausdance, 1993.
Morris, D., *Man Watching.* Jonathan Cape Ltd., London, 1977.
Portnoy, J., *Music in the Life of Man.* Holt, Rinehart and Winston, New York, Chicago, San Francisco, Toronto, London, 1968.
Sherborne, V., *Developmental Movement for Children.* Cambridge University Press, Cambridge, England, 1990.

Sherborne, V., *Building Bridges* and *Good Companions.* (Videorecordings) 1982, distributed by Concord Video, Ipswich, Suffolk, U.K.

Stolnitz, J., *Aesthetics and the Philosophy of Art Criticism.* Houghton Mifflin, Boston, 1960.

NAME INDEX

97

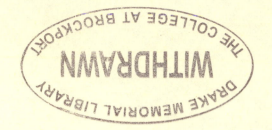